THE
WAY
THROUGH
CHRONIC
PAIN

Tools
To
Reclaim
Your
Healing
Power

ELIZABETH R. KIPP

Publisher
Elizabeth Kipp Media, LLC
900 Massachusetts St. STE 500
Lawrence, KS 66044
Elizabeth-Kipp.com

Elizabeth Kipp Media, LLC
Elizabeth R Kipp, BS, RYT/IKYTA, Founder

The term "Ancestral Clearing" is a trademark for the work of John Newton and Health Beyond Belief.

Cover Design
Gregory Cohane

Page Layout
Robert Lanphear, Lanphear Design

Editorial
Robyn M Fritz, Alchemy West, Inc.
Laurel Robinson, Laurel Robinson Editorial Services

Photographer
Catherine Just, Catherine Just Photography

Library of Congress Control Number: 2019912352

ISBN: 978-0-9983511-3-1
ISBN e-book: 978-0-9983511-2-4
ISBN audiobook: 978-0-9983511-1-7

Printed in the United States of America

Dedication

After I'd spent more than forty years going to doctors all over the world, looking for health and healing, Dr. Peter Przekop, DO, PhD, was the first one who considered my health situation in terms of my whole self—my mind, body, and spirit. He was a phenomenally gifted healer and a fierce force for love. Those of us who knew him felt the sweet, deep, and indelible mark he left on our hearts. He looked beyond the specific diagnosis and prognosis that many other doctors had given me. He stared straight into me and saw who I truly was: a being trapped in the grip of chronic pain who was waiting to emerge and experience the healing power tucked inside of me so that I could fully blossom. He opened the door and then guided me into releasing the awesome, powerful potential to heal that lived inside of me. He taught me and thousands of others how to live life free of pain and suffering.

One of the most profound things he taught me was to accept what is. Peter was here on earth teaching us that we don't have to suffer and showing us how to do that—to not suffer. For real.

This book is gratefully and lovingly dedicated to the memory of Dr. Peter Przekop, for his vision of a world free from suffering and for developing a methodology to free chronic pain sufferers from their prison of hopelessness.

This book is dedicated to the countless people—health care workers of all kinds, friends, and family members—who were along for any part of my journey through chronic pain. Your presence and encouragement kept me as physically fit as they could and lifted me in hope when I would otherwise have been lost to depression and hopelessness.

This book is dedicated to the millions of chronic pain sufferers around the globe who are looking for their way through the pain.

Finally, this book is also dedicated to all those who suffered from chronic pain and addiction and never found their way out.

What is chronic pain?

Pain does not distinguish between physical, emotional, or spiritual. It all sends the same signal to the brain: "it hurts."

Chronic pain is any pain that is felt fifteen days out of thirty for three months or more.

Contents

Finding Your Way Through
The Last Undiscovered Country: Facing Yourself
The Battlefield of Chronic Pain: The Mind and Safety
The Unfolding Journey of Healing: The Great Unwinding

Chapter 1
The Limitations of Science
The Limitations of Western Medicine
Where Is the Healing Field?
Our Source of Healing
The Promise of the Healing Field

Chapter 2

Chapter 3
Where Does the Power to Heal Live?
Who Is Responsible for Your Healing?
Willingness
Becoming Curious
When Healing Becomes Unstoppable

Chapter 4
The Example of My Story and the Power of Changing Focus
Time Tripping and Its Contribution to Chronic Pain
The Art of Passing Time
The Mind Trap: How Attention Can Sabotage Us

Blessing

I prayed for clarity and became a visionary.
I prayed for deep listening and felt my pain dissolve.
I prayed for change and learned to accept the moment.
I prayed for connection to You and found my heartbeat.
I prayed to find You and found You everywhere.
I prayed for patience and learned how to surf the
chaotic waves of my life.
I prayed for stillness and found it waiting in the breath.
I prayed for steadiness and found thanksgiving.
I prayed for guidance and found courage to step
into the unknown.
I prayed for peace and learned to forgive all parts of myself.
I prayed for abundance and learned to drop my fears.
I prayed for wealth and riches and found health and well-being.
I prayed to find ease and grace in life,
and I learned to love myself.
I prayed for liberation and found meditation.
I prayed for joy and found its root in gratitude.
I prayed for love and found it when I opened to receive it.
I prayed for a miracle and discovered I was the miracle.
I prayed for my soul mate and found myself.
I prayed for a way out of the darkness and found Your light
surrounding me.
I prayed for protection and found Your love.
I prayed for my purpose and found it in service to You.

Foreword

When I met Elizabeth, it was early in her recovery from chronic pain and addiction, yet it was apparent she was willing to do whatever it took to thrive in her recovery. She sought out my help as a yoga therapist, somatic healer, and counselor, and she enthusiastically became a student of as much wisdom as I could impart to her. She also sought out the medical support of Dr. Peter Przekop, the teachings of Kundalini yoga, other forms of yoga, twelve-step programs, and more.

As she ardently employed various techniques as a student, she also became a gifted sponsor to those practicing the twelve-step lifestyle, a Kundalini yoga teacher, an Ancestral Clearing Practitioner, a Bilateral EFT/Tapping Practitioner, and a health facilitator. Elizabeth has already helped many on their journeys to healing their chronic pain. She has grown deeper in her practice and more committed to her recovery community. It has been an honor for me to have a front row seat where I have listened and helped guide her in her growth. She is now a true woman of wisdom in the chronic pain and addiction recovery world.

Having said all that, I have personally spent more than forty years as a movement and yoga therapist, which has given me the opportunity to work closely with thousands of people who sought out my guidance to feel better and thrive. When I experienced my personal cycles of chronic pain, suffering, and healing, I sought help in many of the same kinds of places Elizabeth did. I also had the privilege of having learned from Elizabeth's journey and wisdom, which helped me heal my chronic pain!

Elizabeth's book on chronic pain is very insightful for the times we are in. We all know about chronic pain either from our own experience or from someone close to us. Any injury, illness, or suffering that occupies our consciousness or keeps us in a cycle of pain for more than a few weeks is considered chronic. The protocols that have been prescribed or guided by our medical professionals or even our close relations all too often further our suffering. Whether it be the inappropriate use of opioids or the attempts to distract us from our sufferings, we may be temporarily relieved but are rarely healed.

Elizabeth presents a new perspective that all addictions, whether to food, gambling, sex, drugs, or alcohol, represent the many faces of chronic pain. This simplified understanding of addiction is very helpful for what is required to succeed at recovery.

The greatest challenge has always been healing the addictive habits that hold people to their cycles of suffering. As patterns of the body and mind organize, the brain directs our mind's interactions with the world. When we move, think, breathe, and act in suffering, we tend to stay in suffering.

How to break the patterns of suffering is well presented in Elizabeth's adventure in healing. Elizabeth takes us on a rare journey through the mind of a scientist. As a trained academic, she presents a scientific study of herself through her years of traumas, addictions, and suffering. We are invited to join her on a study of the anatomy and physiology of a miracle. All recoveries from chronic pain and addiction are miraculous, but rarely are we offered such a scientific perspective. The groundwork is laid out here as a path for others to follow. We are given a new picture of addiction as a lifestyle of chronic pain. It is only by healing the chronic pain cycles that we can get to the source of addiction.

This book is a valuable source of inspiration and guidance to better navigate the challenges of chronic pain and addiction. It will provide you with a new understanding of chronic pain from the unique perspective of someone who is both a patient and a scientist. Having the language of both suffering and science is a great aid to our understanding of this epidemic. And it is a gift to have a map of the path to recovery.

Guru Prem Singh Khalsa
Yoga therapist, somatic healer, and in recovery from chronic pain

Preface

I came to a point where I was just done with the pain. I made a decision and a commitment to better myself and do whatever it took to find my way through chronic pain. It wasn't about getting rid of it or getting away from it. It was about finding my way through it. And that's a big distinction when it comes to pain. When we try to get rid of pain or avoid it or even numb it or any of that kind of thing, we're just feeding it. But if we can learn to just sit and accept and surrender to our experience, suddenly that energy changes from the pain of trying to funnel Niagara Falls through a pipe to the pipe just disappearing and you becoming Niagara Falls.

I wrote this book to give chronic pain sufferers a guide through the path of healing. I wrote this book for those in the health care field and for the caretakers and loved ones who work with chronic pain sufferers.

My experience of talking with thousands of chronic pain sufferers is that the voice of chronic pain is misunderstood or not heard at all. In chronic pain, we tend to speak from one of two extremes: either we constantly complain, or we remain silent. I have done my best to honestly give voice to the chronic pain sufferer and to offer the insights I gained from finding my way through chronic pain. If people better understand this terrain, chronic pain sufferers are more likely to get higher-quality help and heal faster.

The body and the breath are always in the present moment, but we chronic pain sufferers go to great lengths to dissociate from what we are feeling physically, emotionally, or spiritually. Our sense of safety is so threatened that we collapse our breath and our self-esteem. Our connection to our friends, our family, ourselves, and our Higher Power is sorely tested, even to the breaking point.

Chronic pain steals our attention away from everything but itself. Our power is greatly diminished as we grapple with the forces it brings to bear. We lose track of the present moment, becoming hooked by our past and harried by what we imagine about our future. Our breath is shortened, so we forget how to relax into the long exhale. When our breathing pattern becomes dysfunctional, we lose our ability to nourish the body. When we dissociate from the body, we vacate the very place where our healing power lies. We leave the body temple, the place where the mind, body, and spirit merge.

Western culture views pain as something to avoid by treating or numbing it or by somehow altering the way we experience it as sensation. I am not saying that we should never use pain medication. However, I am saying that we need to use pain medication wisely. We are at war with pain. We have forgotten that pain is simply a part of healing.

To heal chronic pain and its effects we must reclaim the body temple. It is a journey that at its core is spiritual in nature. We must take back our power from the clutches of chronic pain. We must reconnect to and deepen our relationship with ourselves and with our Higher Power: Source of All That Is, including the source of our healing.

This is the journey I took to reclaim my body temple. Here I trace the steps and share the tools I used to pry myself free from the grip of chronic pain. I rediscovered the peace in being comfortable in my own skin. I reclaimed my power—physical, emotional, and spiritual—to shift from living my fate to living my destiny. And I discovered the power of healing that lives so deeply and dynamically within.

This is the journey you can take, too. Your body wants to heal. You do not have to suffer.

Introduction

*The greatest progress is when you know your limitations
and then you have the courage to drop them.*

— Yogi Bhajan

As of the fall of 2019, I am six years in recovery from more than four decades of chronic pain. To achieve that, I used the tools I am writing about, tools those of us in recovery must use every day for the rest of our lives. They helped me conquer doubt, dread, and despair. Like you, I am just another spirit having a human experience, but I have faith in my experience, and faith in the urgings of my soul to follow this path.

Finding Your Way Through

You have stepped into a larger world, perhaps even a new one for you. Living in chronic pain can feel like you have grabbed a tiger by the tail and cannot remember how to let it go. I know. I am familiar with how this feels, since I lived with chronic pain. Chronic pain is the nightmare roller coaster ride of our life.

You may feel that you have been doomed to live a life ruled—indeed dominated—by suffering chronic pain. I am here to tell you that your situation does not have to be a hopeless one. The body wants to heal. You don't have to suffer.

Consider this example of my client Claire's lived experience:

Claire: "I've looked everywhere. I've seen scores of doctors. I've taken the medicines. I've done what I was told. The medicine isn't working. I am still in pain, and it's getting worse. I'm losing hope. I feel like I am standing on the edge of a ledge and will fall any moment. Surely there is another way to live, one without this constant suffering from chronic pain. Tell me what to do. I'll do it. Just help me, please. You have gone through chronic pain and come out the other side. Can you help me?"

Me: "Yes. I am not a doctor or a therapist. However, I have gone through decades of chronic pain and found help to heal my condition and a way to live a life without suffering. I am happy to teach you the tools that worked for me."

I sat calmly with this chronic pain sufferer. First, I asked Claire to just breathe and drop any struggle with the pain. We talked for a short while, and I listened to Claire's story. She had never been able to tell her story to anyone who truly seemed to hear her. The relief in Claire's voice from finally being heard was palpable. Next, I did an Ancestral Clearing with her.

Claire felt a pronounced shift and release in her pain. "Wow!" she said. "I feel calm and ease in my body. I wasn't sure that this would ever be possible for me again in my life. For the first time in eleven years, I have hope."

Claire's experience is an example of what is possible with chronic pain. The brain is changed by chronic pain. We need to bring modalities that help heal those changes. Opiates and benzodiazepines, often prescribed to treat chronic pain, do not heal the changes that chronic pain imposes on the brain. Doctors are generally not trained in how to heal chronic pain, only in how to help us numb it. There are ways to recover from chronic pain.

This book is about the tools I used to heal chronic pain. You can heal from chronic pain using a mind, body, spirit approach that addresses the whole person. I am proof of that. Let me tell you about it.

Healing from chronic pain is a process. You won't find a pill to heal it. But you already knew that, didn't you? You're searching for a life free from the pain of suffering, a life that allows you to fulfill the promise of your best self—the one you came here to live.

The solution to the enigma of chronic pain lies in changing our perspective on, and our approach to, the problem of pain. When we look at the problem chronic pain sets before us, we find the solution to it in its very nature.

It is important to understand that you have done nothing wrong. Too often, we sufferers of this condition feel we are somehow at fault for it. Our self-esteem falters. The human body is a finely tuned instrument honed over countless generations to endure at least long enough to reproduce. Our nervous system is designed to react to stimuli in our environment so that we survive regardless of the adversity we encounter. We come equipped with a powerful threat assessment system that moves us toward safety. In people who are chronically stressed, this system becomes dysregulated and we feel we are constantly under threat. The whole body is doing all it can to handle the effects of stress. So, understand that your chronic pain situation is an adaptive behavior, however maladjusted it is to your current reality.

Chronic pain is a disease of the brain. You may feel the sensation of pain somewhere in the body, but it is the brain's perception that is driving the sensation you are feeling. The way chronic pain changes the brain sheds light on its solution. The brain becomes chaotic, restive, and hypervigilant, problems that show up as difficulty with memory, focus, sleeping, and impulse control.

A chronic pain sufferer experiences higher levels of anxiety and depression because of the insidiously negative bias in the brain. Since chaos reigns in the brain of chronic pain sufferers, modalities that bring ease and peace are effective in healing such changes. In a nutshell, when we bring calmness back into the system through the mind, body, and spirit, we have direct access to healing chronic pain. It's that simple, though it takes diligence and commitment to effect such healing. Since we are making a lifestyle change, the tools that conquer chronic pain must be used daily.

These steps to wellness define the path to clearing the chaotic reactivity caused by chronic pain. These are the steps you need to take to heal:

- Be willing to see things differently. Change your perspective . . . and stop judging the pain . . . and yourself.
- Stop resisting the pain.
- If you are taking opiates and/or benzodiazepines for your chronic pain, detox off them with the help of a trained professional.
- Eat a healthy, anti-inflammatory diet, and hydrate!
- Clear your ancestral burden, both in your lineage and in your past.
- Learn meditation and other embodied healing practices to quiet the mind and give your nervous system a chance to heal.
- Be committed to your healing.
- Love yourself fiercely and without reservation.
- Do the work to heal: one day at a time for the rest of your life.
- Be grateful.

The Last Undiscovered Country: Facing Yourself

Ultimately, this book is about facing yourself, since the power to heal lives inside you.

With willingness and honesty, you will be able to go within yourself and do the self-awareness work to retrain habits that have kept you in the cycle of suffering. You can unleash your healing power by shifting these habits from counterproductive and even destructive to productive ones.

This work is about learning to "be" rather than "do."

Most of the work here is not thinking-type work. As people suffering from chronic pain, we are often hijacked by our thoughts because of what the pain does to the body's entire nervous system. We want to figure out what is causing the constant pain. We want to find another doctor, therapist, or modality, thinking maybe this next one will be the answer. We want to control what is happening to us. I understand. I was one of those people. I am *not* advocating that you stop looking for an answer. However, this book does not address that. Rather, it encourages self-discovery.

This teaching was passed down to me through many other teachers. They pointed me right back into myself, just as their teachers did for them. I discovered so much inside myself: so much waiting to be healed, so much healing power, and more.

These are all available to you.

May you find as I did that your great undiscovered country is the one that lives inside you. May you come to realize, as I have, how vast that country is and the inner peace that lives there deep in the center. As the center of the hurricane is a place of still and quietude, so is that place within yourself. May you find that no matter how chaotic the winds of life become, you always have that place of stillness to ground yourself in the center of your being.

The Battlefield of Chronic Pain: The Mind and Safety

Fear thrives in the mind.

Where is the mind? This is a question that has been asked for thousands of years. Currently, we are learning that "the mind" can be found in the brain, the heart, the vagus nerve, and the gut. My view is that when we view the human organism as a whole being, the mind is everywhere in the body.

As chronic pain sufferers, we get taken down by our pain. As its captive, we become its victim. We are intensely challenged. For us to really deal with this situation, we must understand where this struggle is taking place. We have long realized that we are on the battlefield, but few of us realize that the war zone is the mind, which comprises not only our thoughts but the underlying physiology that drives those thoughts.

How do we begin to address this? What is our strategy, and what tactics will we use?

It is important to remember that our perception of our safety is at the root of all our reactivity to pain. We feel uncomfortable. Our intricate nervous system has perceived a threat, whether internal or external, and is reacting in a way that causes us to act to preserve ourselves. Because chronic pain sufferers feel threatened all the time, their nervous system, their "mind," is in a state of constant reactivity and defense. They are using only part of the brain, the part that reverts to a protective mode, rather than being able to access it in a fully integrated way. The strategy, then, is to bring balance back into "the mind" through the nervous system with embodied practices that help reset the entire system so that it is fully cohesive and united.

Let's look at a larger view. We may feel like we are isolated, but we are not alone in the suffering. Although each of us must face our individual mind states alone, it is important to understand that we are not alone in this dilemma. One out of every four people in just the United States experiences chronic pain. We can find some help by joining with others in sharing our experience, strength, and hope on healing from this malady.

To heal chronic pain, we need to summon our courage and meet the challenge. We have lost our sense of wholeness, in mind, body, and spirit. We have lost the sense of divine alignment between ourselves and our innate healing power, and the present moment—what I call the Healing Field.

We must rise above our victimhood and become unafraid of the pain. Fear thrives in our thoughts. We have sensation in the body, and it can be intense. We feel it, and then our thoughts come in and create a story about what we are feeling. The chronic pain sufferer often makes a judgment call that what they are feeling is "bad," and so the battle of our thoughts versus "pain" begins.

Next, we lose track of the present moment as we access the past for reference and then project into our future, based on what happened to us. We conclude that our sense of safety is threatened. We start resisting the pain. We start pushing against it. We try to control it. Then the pain pushes back in at least equal measure. We push harder and try harder to control it. The pain pushes harder, meeting us with the force we bring to it. The more we fight, the farther we move out of the Healing Field.

And so, the cycle of suffering begins. So long as this conflict remains, the pain is the one in control. Thus, we are suddenly and seemingly inextricably in the throes of all-out warfare with the pain. We have given our power away to the pain and to this conflict. Our access to the Healing Field is blocked. We get trapped here in suffering. It is all taking place inside "the mind."

This book will help you regain your alignment with the principles that give you access to the Healing Field and bring this internal war to a peaceful end.

The Unfolding Journey of Healing:
The Great Unwinding

The journey to healing is one that unfolds. Much as we may want to, there is no rushing this process. It happens in its own time. Our best move is to do what we can to feed, water, exercise, and rest the body, learn to handle the mind's habits, and allow the healing process to happen. We can encourage it, but any attempt on our part to control it will only serve to get in the way of the healing process itself.

We live in a culture of instant gratification. Life is fast paced. We are up against deadlines and can feel pushed to "make things happen." Indeed, a motivating cheer I hear today in personal development and leadership forums is "Make it happen!" I am all for taking action steps; however, our healing space is not the place for this kind of energy. We cannot force the process. We nurture it and accept the rhythm of the power of healing. The innate wisdom inside us knows the path. Healing is not a linear but an organic process that follows its own meanderings. It is our job is to allow the path to reveal itself to us.

Imagine that you are in a rose garden you have just planted. It is early spring, and you have planted bare root rosebushes, painstakingly covering them with loamy soil rich in organic matter and liberally watering them. You are so excited about your new garden! You watch the bushes develop young green shoots and expand into branches filled with beautiful green leaves. You marvel at the vigorous life force expressing itself through these plants.

One day you notice that pink flower buds have sprouted all over the new bushes. You anticipate the thought of the heady fragrances that are soon to lace the air with sweetness. You are so intent on smelling the essence of rose that you lose all patience and proceed to open a developing rose blossom. But you discover that it does not have that wondrous smell you were anticipating. In your push to rush the growing process, you ended up getting in the way of it.

This is what we do with our healing when we anticipate and judge how it will be. We must understand and remind ourselves that we aren't doing the healing. We are doing what we can to help the healing move along, and ideally not rushing the process. The problem with trying to rush is that we end up standing in healing's way, much like when we tried to rush the rose blossom into unfolding before its time.

My experience has shown me that healing from chronic pain is a process of unwinding. It takes time for us to develop the syndrome of chronic pain and the consequent changes in the mind, body, and soul. It takes time for us to unwind it and for the brain to heal. It takes time to regain our sense of safety and re-regulate the nervous system to normal. We are doing mind, body, and soul work here, so we are healing on all fronts.

I observed that the longer I hurt, the more I wound myself up in tension. It was as if I were a giant toy top, getting wound up little by little but most assuredly tighter and tighter. In my recovery, I have noticed a gradual uncoiling of tension inside me. I get a little calmer each day. I feel as if I am journeying down a long road that is unwinding in front of me. It is not a straight road. It has its own twists and turns, valleys and hills, and it is always outstretched before me, beckoning me forward.

Doctors can clean a wound, stitch the torn skin together, and give us orders to help optimize our healing, but it is the body that holds the mysterious and profound healing power. Your healing will happen in perfect time and right on schedule, although perhaps maybe not the way you expect. And herein lies one of the great lessons healing brings us: patience.

Give yourself a break. Love yourself and bow to the mystery living inside of you. It is divine energy that is directing the whole show. Once you have paid your entrance fee by doing the work needed to set the best conditions, you can sit back and allow your healing miracle to unfold.

1

The Healing Field

*The promise of the Healing Field is the discovery
of your innate healing power.*

— Elizabeth Kipp

The Limitations of Science

Science is self-limiting. Science can observe, describe, and quantify. However, science cannot solve or explain why: it can only point us in the direction of a solution. The framework of the scientific model is restricted to phenomena that are observable and can be described or quantified.

Science works with probabilities. Experimental data shows us that under certain conditions, an event is likely to occur. The occurrence of that event is not a hard rule every time the event happens, but an expectation based on observational data and statistics. We can analyze the frequency of past events and make a guess, forecasting the probability that a certain event will occur. It is a guess. Often it is a good guess, but it remains a guess. My understanding of this inherent principle of science was foundational to understanding what Western medicine, based solely in the realm of science, can and cannot bring to the table when it comes to healing.

The Limitations of Western Medicine

Chronic pain creates chaos and a marked negative bias in the brain. It steals our attention, making it difficult to focus. It disturbs our sleep cycle and fundamentally upsets our internal balance. Chronic pain is a condition brought about by mind, body, and spiritual dissonance.

Western doctors are not routinely trained in how to treat chronic pain. They are taught to use the pharmaceutical option as the standard course of treatment, though that is beginning to change in some clinics.

Opiates and benzodiazepines have not been found to heal chronic pain and can exacerbate the problem by adding addiction to pain.

The line from the Hippocratic Oath "First, do no harm" is on shaky ground when a chronic pain patient is prescribed opioid medications to treat the pain. These medications become less effective over time. Opioid pain medications have powerfully unhealthy side effects. They bring the digestive system to a state of paralysis, so that a body trying to heal can neither take in nutrients effectively nor release toxic waste products. Opiates are also dehydrating, and so, once again, the body has a more difficult job cleaning itself as it tries to heal the underlying cause of the chronic pain. Opiates also cause hyperalgesia, which makes the pain worse instead of helping to heal it. Use of these medications shows there is no progress toward solving the problem of chronic pain, which is caused by the nonalignment and disconnection of mind, body, and spirit.

Where Is the Healing Field?

The Healing Field lives in the present moment. We cannot heal in the past or the future. We can only heal in the here and now. However, when we're in chronic pain, we tend to link our pain to our past experience and project our fears about our pain into the future. We miss the present moment altogether, and so bypass the only healing space available to us.

Our Source of Healing

We are trying to solve an integration problem in healing from chronic pain. We have lost our way to the Healing Field, where we become aware of the merger of body, mind, and spirit. Perhaps this all seems like a riddle. We may have thought we had a health problem that was rooted in a physical ailment. But if it were that simple, we would have healed long ago, and chronic pain would not even be on our radar.

In the final analysis, we feel distinctly repelled by our condition. We may even be angry or feel utterly let down by our concept of a Higher Power. Maybe we feel we are being punished. However it plays out, we feel disconnected from our Creator, maybe to the point of feeling abandoned. Our work to heal our chronic pain must include healing the chasm between ourselves and our Higher Power.

The pain itself, whether physical, emotional, or psychological, boils down to being spiritual in nature. We do not accept what we are experiencing in the present moment. We long for something else. We long for release from the grip of chronic pain. We long for freedom. In all this longing, we never find relief. We long for something that we perceive is in the future, and so have not yet accepted our present experience.

The need to fill this longing inside us is at the root of the pain. The longing itself presents as a void with an endless bottom. No matter what we turn to—food, electronics, people and relationships, money, shopping, drugs . . . no matter what we try, the longing remains. Our search reaps nothing but more seeking, more pain, and more suffering.

We hear in spiritual circles that we need to "look within." What does that mean, and how do we do it in practice?

First, recognize that what you have been doing so far has not been working. Then consider making a different choice and taking a contrary action. Instead of looking "out there" to fill the longing—the great void you feel inside—look within yourself.

How do you do that?

Learn to live in the present moment. Learn to accept your feelings—all of them.

For instance, when you next feel the longing, simply sit with it instead of trying to fill it with something. Here, in the present moment, you enter the Healing Field. Release your judgment about your experience. Drop your resistance to being with the longing. Accept your experience. Get curious instead of fearful of what might be waiting for you in this experience. Sit quietly and watch what happens. Release any expectation of an outcome and remain in the spirit of inquiry.

This is a spiritual exercise in faith. Tap into your courage and take a great leap of faith when you allow yourself to accept whatever may arise within this space of longing and this seemingly unfillable void that lives inside you.

This space can seem like a great mystery. As chronic pain sufferers, we have spent so much of our lives dodging this place that the present moment is not well known to us.

Let me remind you that spiritual teachers have been saying for ages that the creation of the world, the universe, began as a void. The void is the birthplace of all creation. Embrace the void within. It is as essential a part of you as the universe itself. The longing that lives in this place is really a longing to create. It may seem mysterious to you because its very nature is one of uncertainty. This is a source of connection, of merging with our Higher Power. It is a place to welcome with open arms.

In your search to fill the longing, you just turned in the wrong direction to fulfill it. The experience of the longing is the answer to quenching the thirst we have, this fundamental craving that wants to be sated. The answer was in you all along. When you are finally able to connect with this place inside yourself, you will find that you have at last solved the riddle of the void. You have found your way into the Healing Field. You have found your fountain of creativity. This is a place of spontaneous evolution.

Healing your chronic pain is just one of the outcomes for you when you tap into this internal creative force. Ultimately, you are doing soul-healing work here.

The Promise of the Healing Field

Here is the promise of the Healing Field:

- A solution to chronic pain
- An end to suffering
- The discovery of your innate healing power
- The answer to reintegration and realignment of mind, body, and spirit
- Contentment, peace, and ease in your life

Science and Western medicine cannot fully address the Healing Field, since healing happens both within and outside of the scientific framework. We live in the All That Is; science operates only within the part of the All That Is that it can observe, describe, and measure. We limit our healing potential by referencing our healing only within science. The Creator with its power within us is the ultimate healer. This is not a wishy-washy answer. It is one that comes from science's inability to address the real underlying issue. You can address this issue in yourself.

2

My Experience and Way Through Chronic Pain

As a child I was not given the tools
for handling the stresses in my life.

— Elizabeth Kipp

I grew up in a family that had all the trimmings of success, yet was rife with an undercurrent of uneasiness. The world had just come out of a war that threatened to engulf us all in darkness. Fear ran rampant: it was palpable throughout the family and the culture. Cigarettes and alcohol were the preferred de-stressors for adults. These substances were so common and accepted that my mother continued smoking and consuming alcoholic beverages during her pregnancies with my brother and me.

The "bar" opened at the stroke of five o'clock every evening. My parents and their friends called themselves social drinkers. I never saw them falling-down drunk, yet they used alcohol and occasional doctor-prescribed calming medications to deal with stress. Fortunately, these "coping strategies" were out my reach as a child. I was not given any tools for handling the stresses and strains in my life. I managed the best I could.

We had clearly understood but unwritten and unspoken house rules in both our family and the extended culture. Anything distressing or uncomfortable was not discussed. We didn't look at the invisible "elephant in the room." As children, we were to stay quiet until spoken to. We were told that if we had nothing nice to say, we should be silent. We were not allowed to show emotion, and if we did, we were sorely reprimanded and more. When we did not observe the house rules, we were subject to severe disciplinary measures (abuse). These rules were nonnegotiable.

I was left to my own devices to cope with the stresses of life. I picked up some adaptive behaviors that helped me survive in the short term but were unhealthy in the long term. I kept myself safe by muting cries of pain. I held my emotions inside me. I pushed through whatever I experienced and denied the effects such trauma had on me. No one knew it at the time, but I was already a chronic pain sufferer.

I lived with an almost constant pain in my gut. No one seemed to know the cause. They gave it a name—irritable bowel syndrome—and gave me medication when the pains became intolerable and stopped me in my tracks. I learned to live with a general "low" level of pain.

An underlying principle within the family and culture was that one should learn how to deal with life's pains by pushing through them. The expression "no pain, no gain" echoed throughout my childhood and into adulthood.

At age fourteen, I fell off a horse and landed on my low back on a rock, splitting my fifth lumbar vertebra in two. I knew I had taken a blow, but because I was able to get up and walk, I assumed I was okay. I had a very sore back for about two weeks. The pain in my back felt like the low-level pain in my gut, so I just went on with life.

In 1969, I experienced a profound emotional trauma that went untreated. This only added to my stress.

I went on to finish high school and started college as a sociology major. I enjoyed the sciences so much that I ended up getting a degree in plant science. I married and went to graduate school.

In 1975, I came home from work one day and had difficulty climbing the stairs to my bedroom. That's when I knew I needed medical help. I scheduled appointments with different kinds of doctors who treated back pain. The first one was a chiropractor, who took an X-ray and told me I had an old injury in the lower part of my spine. As soon as he said that, I knew exactly what injury he was referring to. The X-ray revealed that my fifth lumbar had split into two pieces, side to side at the transverse processes, and the front part had slipped forward 25 percent off the spinal column and into my pelvis, pulling the nerves to the legs with it.

The chiropractor said he could help me. All the other doctors told me I needed spinal fusion surgery. I opted for the nonsurgical route, which served me well for another seven years. I had pain, but the chiropractor's adjustments helped keep it tolerable. I didn't take any medication. I rested when I needed to and tried to stay as physically fit as possible.

Then in 1982, nine months after my son's birth, this lumbar area in my spine became unstable, and the orthopedic doctors grew concerned for my continued safety. Concerned that the front part of the vertebra would slip farther off the pelvis and cripple me, they strongly suggested a spinal fusion to stabilize the slip. Even my chiropractor agreed.

I went ahead with the surgery. Coming out of it, my journey with chronic pain skyrocketed to a whole other level. I was given opiates and benzodiazepines to cope with postsurgical pain. The pain now really pulled my attention into it. The medications helped me focus elsewhere so I could concentrate on a task at hand, yet the pain remained a force to be reckoned with.

I had a second surgery just over a year later. This time they tried a different approach to the fusion: Luque rod fixtures set into the bone from the fourth lumbar vertebra to the first sacral level, along with another bone fusion at the fourth and fifth lumbar joint. After the surgery, my pain level increased, and I continued using opiates and benzodiazepines. At this point I was becoming frustrated with the answers I kept getting around pain control. Here we had this medication that could numb pain, but the doctors gave me only enough to take the edge off the sensations I was feeling. "We don't want you to get addicted," they said.

The doctors told me I would be in pain 24/7 for the rest of my life and in a wheelchair by the time I turned forty. Because of my background in the sciences, I realized these pronouncements were inaccurate and potentially harmful. The statements were given as factual outcomes of my condition, but the doctors had forgotten a foundational piece of science: in this realm, we work in probabilities, not in hard and fast "facts."

I also realized that the medical world I had enlisted to help me was limited by its own scientific framework. Science is limited because it must be able to somehow measure the phenomena that it studies—yet we live in an unlimited universe. Once I remembered this, I realized that my healing power was within me, as part of the universe. The doctors could do their part in stabilizing the slip in my spine, but it was my body that was doing the healing. That is, the medical community helped set the circumstances for healing to the best of their ability. I could enlist their expertise and knowledge, but then I had to do everything in my power to effect my own healing.

The front part of the dislodged fifth lumbar slipped to 80 percent of the way into my pelvis, so I had a third spinal fusion in 1986 to stabilize this area. An incisional hernia repair surgery followed in 1988. My pain situation continued to escalate, and my doctor put me on extensive bed rest. I spent six of the years in the 1980s in bed.

The 1990s ushered in a new paradigm for pain control: "We will give you as much opiates and benzodiazepines as we safely can to help you with your pain. We don't care about addiction." I was never quite clear on what forces helped shift this line of thinking, but I experienced it in both Canada and the United States. I lived in both countries during the 1980s and 1990s. It was interesting to see this paradigm operating in both countries.

I continued to look for a solution to my pain beyond this numbing medication route. I worked many different modalities, from acupuncture to massage therapy, energy work, yoga, meditation, and more. My husband, who was also well studied in biological sciences, joined me in doing as much research as we could on the problem of chronic pain. The only solutions we came across dealt with how to treat the pain with medication. The underlying assumption was that people who had chronic pain would always have it, and the only option was to medicate with opiates and benzodiazepines.

I had moments of relief, and then the pain would return and bring me to my knees. I felt as if I were a buoy being tossed around in a turbulent sea, never knowing which way the waters would push me. So, my sense of uncertainty grew along with escalating pain levels. My anxiety increased and transformed into panic attacks. My doctors continued to prescribe stronger and stronger doses of opiates and benzodiazepines. By the time I went into treatment to detox, I was on fentanyl patches, fentanyl quick-acting lollipops, and high doses of Ativan. I was on fentanyl combined with one benzodiazepine or another for fifteen years.

I was so sick all the time that I really felt the medication was contributing to my pain problem as well as my quality-of-life problem. The prescribing doctor did not have a plan to help me withdraw from the medication beyond putting me in a coma while my body detoxed. Given that he had limited experience with this method, I passed on that exit route.

My son reached out to a friend who knew Dr. Peter Przekop, affectionately known as "Dr. P," and had him call me. Dr. P was the director of the Pain Management Program at the Betty Ford Center. I remember him saying, "Maybe your pain medicine is causing some of your pain," and "We can reset your stress response," and "I've helped thousands of people come off opiates and benzos, including fentanyl." I was surprised to hear him say opiates could cause pain. I later learned he was referring to hyperalgesia, a condition about which nothing was published until 2010. I was also surprised that he knew without asking that I had panic attacks.

I decided to go into Dr. P's Pain Management Program. I entered that program with a lifetime of chronic gut pain (fifty-nine years), forty years of back pain, and thirty-two years of taking opiates and benzodiazepines. I experienced a miracle beyond my imagining when I walked out of the program fifty-two days later, free of medication and pain-free.

Dr. P looked at the chronic pain problem from a different perspective than other doctors. His view was that the body had the power to heal, and we just needed to create the optimal conditions in the body so that healing could occur. He knew that chronic pain sufferers contributed to their own suffering. He knew about the changes the brain undergoes with both chronic pain and addiction medications.

Dr. P and his colleagues in the program gave the participants a set of stress management tools and told us we would have to use them every day for the rest of our lives if we were to live a life beyond chronic pain. I gratefully accepted these tools.

After fifty-two days in Dr. P's program, my pain, after so many years, had disappeared. I went into recovery using his tools and learned more helpful lifestyle changes I could make to improve the quality of my life and find stability.

A final note here: until I met Dr. P, the doctors were focused on helping me numb or otherwise dampen my pain experience. Although I had a short daily meditation practice, I spent most of my time remembering my past pain, worrying about pain being in my future, or resenting the pain I was feeling in the present moment. I had not understood the Healing Field and its power, nor had these doctors. Part of the healing that Dr. P helped his patients achieve was the ability to be in the present moment and release judgment about our experience of it.

I am proof that these methods work. And my clients are proof. This path is open to you should you care to walk it.

(3)

Mindset Is Key

You must be willing to believe more in the power of healing than in the power of illness.

— Elizabeth Kipp

Your mindset is a crucial component of healing chronic pain. Your best thinking got you to where you are in your suffering. Start looking from a new perspective. It is time to take stock and consider changing the strategy you have been using. Your openness to questioning your way of doing things and the willingness and courage to try something new are keys to a healthy mindset.

Here are the basic action steps to a healthy mindset. When you implement these actions, your healing will become unstoppable.

- Decide you have had enough.
- Become determined and willing to change and to try new things. You are an active participant in your healing.
- Commit to your healing. Take responsibility for your healing journey.
- Become willing to change your approach to living.
- Say yes to your experience.
- Turn within and open your inner eyes and ears to the Infinite Healer inside you.
- Become curious.
- Be willing to drop the habit of thinking all the time, and spend more time being.

Mindset is at least half of healing. Feed, water, exercise, and rest the body, but if you are to heal and stay healthy, you must also keep a healthy mindset.

Here is what that means. Start with determination and commitment. Your healing begins with you. You can turn to health care professionals for help, but your healing begins with your commitment. Become determined to rise out of pain. I asked myself when I was suffering from chronic pain, and I ask my clients now: What is your commitment to your healing? Are you done with the suffering? Will you go to any lengths to heal?

Where Does the Power to Heal Live?

Your healing power lives within your body. There's nothing wrong with your body: it is simply responding to the world it is living in. Where you can, you need to change the stimulus you are giving it. The first step is realizing where the power to your healing resides: within your body. This is how you unleash your healing power.

It is critical that you own your healing power, because the body wants to heal. It has amazing powers to heal. It has an almost unlimited pharmacy within to manufacture the compounds it needs. First, you must be committed to your healing and learn to look to the wisdom within you.

Many of us are used to putting our health in the hands of the external world, ceding responsibility to doctors and other practitioners in the medical arena. I was raised to do this. Our whole culture has the same mentality. When we get sick, we say, "It's up to them to heal me." Let's get the power structure straight. Doctors can stitch up a wound, but they cannot tell the body how to heal. Only the body knows how to heal. The power to heal lives within you.

Who Is Responsible for Your Healing?

The rule I use for what the healing power structure looks like is that we take 80 percent of the responsibility for our healing and give the other 20 percent to the health care community. The scientific community has great insight into our health and can help us in many ways, but it does not hold the healing power itself. It has limitations. The limitation in science, the foundation of medical knowledge in the Western world, is the framework in which science operates. The design of scientific inquiry and its requirement for measurables restricts the number and types of questions it can answer.

Science works in probabilities, not, as we often believe, in black or white "facts." Things are not as certain as we think they are. It is in the uncertainty that the power to shift our lives resides. Here's what I mean:

We are made up of atoms. Atoms are in a constant state of motion, and depending on the speed of those atoms, things appear as a solid, liquid, or gas. It gets even more magnificent. Physicists have determined that the path of an electron around the nucleus of an atom can be predicted about 95 percent of the time. This gives us an observable electron cloud that is a "reality" we can count on—most of the time. There is, however, that other 5 percent when the electron deviates from the predictable path and we are unable to track it.

Science and the medical world can predict what might happen 95 percent of the time, at best. Hope lives in the other 5 percent.

In addition, since science operates within a strict framework of measurables, it is limited. We live in both the scientific world and the rest of the universe. We live in the All That Is. Our healing lives both in the world of science and outside of it. So it is with your healing.

Your world is only "your world" 95 percent of the time. New possibilities arise without any effort on your part to allow for change. This is the realm we might be tempted to call "magic."

This is the realm where shifts and changes in your healing can happen spontaneously. It is in that 5 percent place where the unpredictable occurs that the field of possibility lies. This is where the transformation lives.

As a chronic pain sufferer used to the conditions you have endured, you must unlearn your old patterning around your reaction to and beliefs about chronic pain. Instead of being locked into your old ways of living in negativity, open yourself to new possibilities. Train yourself to be aware of your reactions, to notice and shift your negativity to a more positive state, and to bring more consciousness into your way of living.

Willingness

You will find yourself coming to a point of surrender with your suffering from chronic pain and its dis-ease. You have had enough. You will do whatever it takes to heal. But you were not always this way. As a chronic pain sufferer, you tend to want to be anywhere but "here" with the pain. You are not comfortable with how you feel. You may notice that you judge how you feel as "bad" and you fear it is how you feel. You may look everywhere but inside yourself for a solution. To heal, you must return to your inner world, to the infinite wisdom that lives within you. Become curious about what may be revealed to you as you listen. Be willing to be present to your experience, no matter what is happening. Become willing to open your inner ears and listen to the words of the soul, where the wisdom to your healing lies.

You must be willing to believe more in the power of healing than in the power of illness.

Your willingness is the beginning of your commitment to heal. It is a powerful start. Become willing to say yes to what is happening, rather than trying to avoid it, numb it, or make it disappear.

This place of saying yes to our experience was pivotal for me. I spent years trying to change my circumstances, to fix them.

This strategy only kept me going in the same direction of pain and more pain. When I became willing, I learned to accept my experience instead of fighting it.

Physics reveals to us that an object will remain at rest or stay in motion until acted on by an outside force. To heal chronic pain, you need to change the direction of its motion. You must act in a way contrary to how you have been acting. Instead of turning away from your pain, the contrary action is to turn into it. Instead of trying to get away from your body, the contrary action is to turn into and go deeply into your body. Become an inner explorer. You will realize when you go within yourself that the great undiscovered country lives there. You will discover the healing power that you have held all along but has eluded you.

These concepts around willingness will most likely be nebulous and not fully understood until you put them into action. You must have the *experience* of surrendering, of saying yes, of changing the trajectory of your motion. Until you have done this, the concept of willingness is just that: a concept. You need to make it a reality.

Becoming Curious

Once you have developed the ability to say yes to your experience, you can take the next step toward becoming a curious observer of yourself. Begin to ask, *What are the beliefs I have about my pain?*

For example, *Do I believe "something is wrong" with me?* Or, *Do I believe I am "broken"? Do I say to myself, I don't know if I will ever get better?* Perhaps you say to yourself, *I will always be like this, so I will somehow find a way around it.*

What do you believe about the possibilities for change? What assumptions are you making about your condition? Are they true? Are you willing to change your approach?

When you can shift your beliefs about your limitations, you open yourself to a whole new realm of possibility for your healing.

Get curious about expanding beyond your limitations. Ask yourself, *Who am I without my pain?* Perhaps you have been in pain so long that you don't know who you would be without it. It's okay *not* to know. Get curious about not knowing.

When Healing Becomes Unstoppable

Because the brain becomes chaotic in chronic pain, we experience confusion. To heal the brain, we must quiet the mind. The state of being, experienced through the practice of mindfulness, calms the mind and allows the nervous system to reset to normal through the healing process.

The power of presence in and of itself as a healing tool cannot be overstated. When you interrupt the frenetic defensiveness in the nervous system with rest and healing, you change its momentum.

Allow yourself to pause. Allow for the possibility that there is another state of being outside the chaos you have been experiencing. Presence opens you. There is no burden from the past, no expectation of the future. There is only now.

All the energy your thoughts create about any story drops away. There is only the energy of the moment. You tap straight into the heart of healing. By quieting your thoughts, you get them out of the way so that the body can then go about its miraculous power to heal. When you access this space, you effect such a shift that your healing becomes unstoppable.

4

Attention: The Shift from Angst to Peace

When you feel you're at the end of your rope, tie a knot and climb back up.

— Tiffany Farmer

Where our attention is focused when we experience chronic pain can make the difference between feeling angst and feeling peace. Depending on how we use it, attention is a super-tool that can help us heal and clear chronic pain.

Many of us spend most if not all our time in our thoughts. We ignore, distract, or numb ourselves from what we are feeling in our body. These are favorite tactics of chronic pain sufferers. The danger here is that we can end up being at the beck and call of our thoughts instead of making more conscious decisions about how we engage with them. Ideally, we want to have our thoughts in hand, not reigning over us.

When our attention remains on our thoughts and we have pain, we ignore the bodily sensation and feed the story our thoughts create about our pain. We are not feeling the body. We are not feeling the sensations that accompany chronic pain, whether its source is physical, emotional, psychological, or spiritual in nature. Yet in its intelligence, the body is trying to heal, so it increases the intensity of the signal it is giving us. The body is trying to get our attention to get our help in the healing process. The more we ignore, distract from, or numb out this signal, the stronger the body will react to ensure its signal gets through to our consciousness. This cycle can continue a repeating loop unless we act to interfere with it. The focus of our attention is such a tool.

The Example of My Story and the Power of Changing Focus

The only way to beat the mind at its own game is to stop playing.

— John Newton

Here's an example of what can happen when we keep our attention on our thoughts and stay disassociated from the body, a common strategy for chronic pain sufferers. I have met many other chronic pain sufferers who share my experience.

For most of my life, I felt restless. No matter how much I exercised, I still felt edgy. I never found deep peace. My mind was also restless. It took me all over the map—its map, that is. Not knowing how to get a handle on its proclivities, I felt subject to its whimsies and turmoil. My attention was scattered; I perceived that I had no control over the chaotic nature of my mind. I felt unsettled in mind and body.

I had another practice, one far more dangerous. Whenever I sensed an uncomfortable feeling in my body, I ignored it. I didn't want to feel it, and deep down I was threatened by it. My feelings seemed so strong that I felt like I would lose control over my body if I fully felt them. And since no one ever spoke about this, I thought it was just something I was dealing with by myself.

I took that powerful tool of attention and turned it promptly *away from* any uncomfortable feeling. Unless I was brought to my knees, or stopped cold in my tracks by pain, I just kept refocusing my attention away from physical or emotional pain to get away from it, to escape from its grip on me. I ignored it and then "pushed through" whatever circumstance I was experiencing at the time.

I could never quite put my finger on the source of these internal feelings of pressured energy. Unable to silence the underlying tensions by just imagining them into submission, I took up meditation. I learned how to use my attention to laser focus on one sound and allow my thoughts to parade into and out of my mind. But I unknowingly misapplied this tool. Even during meditation, I felt underlying tension. I kept trying to outwit the myriad thoughts I was having, which turned out to be a losing proposition.

In time, I realized that turning away from my physical pain was not helping to decrease it, so I tried using my focusing ability *on* the pain as a possible answer. Interestingly, when I *turned toward* the physical pain I was experiencing and allowed myself to drop my resistance to it and feel the pain fully, I found that the pain itself receded—not all the way, but significantly.

This focusing helped bolster the effect of the pain medications, but none of these things took all the pain away. And I had to have my attention fully on the pain and drop my resistance to it before I felt it subside. Once my attention moved on to something else, the magnitude of the pain returned. This was as close as I got to finding my own answer to my tension. It was a big clue, but I needed more direction before I could fully experience the superpower that the tool of attention really could be.

As time passed and I kept ignoring these uncomfortable feelings, I developed intense physical pain. I developed such chronic gut and back pain that I lost track of the time in my life when I *didn't* have pain. None of the doctors throughout my life had been able to adequately treat it. Yes, they could shoot me up with a drug to knock out the pain, but that was only a temporary fix. Very temporary—and *not* a solution. Even the best doctors did not seem to have a clue what to do to help me heal from this chronic pain.

Opioid pain medication couldn't quell it. On top of that, my restlessness morphed exponentially into anxiety and panic attacks. My doctors gave me drugs (benzodiazepines) to help control my anxiety. Not only did these medications ultimately not help, but I unwittingly got addicted to them just like I did to the opioids, and they worsened my anxiety and insomnia problems. Thus, the choices I had made to address my restlessness and ignore the discomfort in my body only helped to exponentially grow the problem.

John Newton, one of the practitioners in the Pain Management Program, helped me hone my skills at using the tool of my attention. John spoke about the power of story in our lives, and how much more powerful it was to go deeper than our story. He explained that with every story has an emotional component that is expressed as a sensation in the body, like tightness in the stomach or heat in the chest. Our body is trying to get our attention by giving us these feelings, but instead of putting our attention on the sensations in the body, we tend to go into our thoughts and generate a story about what the feelings mean. Our thoughts both create all kinds of meaning about what we are feeling and judge the whole situation, which is a strategy that can perpetuate the suffering of chronic pain.

"All this story does is feed suffering," I heard John say one day.

Suddenly I had an aha moment: "I've been doing this my whole life!"

I had been doing everything *but* be still and attend to the sensations my body was relaying. I had been feeding the story of my pain with more and more story.

John said, "The only way to beat the mind at its own game is to stop playing."

What a profound statement! This was what I had been seeking for years, a way to move away from the constant thoughts I had about my pain and onto a path that would help calm the chaos I was experiencing.

All I needed to do was direct my attention away from my thoughts and direct it toward what my body was feeling . . . and breathe.

I had understood the part about using the attention, but I had misdirected it. I had been looking to calm my thoughts, but I was going to lose every time. I needed to look to the body. Further, I discovered that there was nothing for me to fear by feeling these sensations. In fact, they were not to be ignored or discarded: they were important communications from my body.

John's guidance was more persistent than my old behavior. Every time I fell back into the old habit of sinking into the grip of a story, John gently guided me back to the sensation in my body. He'd point out, "There's the story again. Drop it and go to the sensation you are feeling in your body. What is the sensation you are feeling?"

Suddenly, the pieces to the puzzle of finding the peace within that had eluded me for years fell into place. I had finally found a way to shift the focus of my attention to where it needed to be. A key realization was that I could turn my attention to my thoughts or my body, but not both at the same time; when I focused on my body, my chattering thoughts dropped out of the equation. With enough practice, I was finally able to adopt this new, healthier behavior into my lifestyle.

As I began properly implementing the tool of attention, the gut pain from irritable bowel syndrome I had experienced for so long began to dissolve. My anxiety dropped from a fever pitch to a dull roar and then to just an undercurrent of tension. There were other modalities and other people who helped me dissolve my chronic pain, but this was certainly a powerful start. I was amazed and almost in disbelief that the pain was disappearing. I felt like I was inhabiting a new body.

You, too, can learn to turn the tool of attention toward whatever you are feeling, become present to it, and allow yourself to fully feel it without resistance. Imagine that you are riding your feeling as a surfer rides an ocean wave. Experience its rise and fall and then its dissolution back into the sea. You may notice that some feelings are stronger than others, requiring you to shift and purposefully breathe as the feeling crests, rolls, and tumbles back into the mists within the ocean of your emotions.

Being present to and simply feeling what you feel inside the body as sensation without judgment allows you to just live in the moment, to let go of any fear of losing control of your feelings. Accept what you are feeling. In your acceptance, you will find a measure of peace.

Time Tripping and Its Contribution to Chronic Pain

We tend to reference the past and try to predict our future. It's a habit—and no wonder. Our ancestors survived for ages by using their memories of past experiences to help them act in the present moment and plan, so we come by this referencing naturally. Of course, we need this ability, but taken to an extreme, it can be a hindrance and hold us in the cycle of chronic pain. We can end up spending so much time in the past or the future that we miss the power of the present moment. When we do this, we end up standing directly in the way of our ability to heal.

Here is an example of how I contributed to my pain by time tripping.

One morning I woke up and felt a tight band of sharp stabbing pain in the back of my neck. I felt muscles all over my body tense in reaction to it. The first thing I remember is hearing myself say, "I remember when I had this pain before." Notice I did two things automatically, reflexively. The only consciousness I brought into the moment was the awareness of my thoughts. First, I labeled the sensation I was feeling "pain" as I recoiled against it. Next, I time-tripped into the past to compare what I was experiencing to a previous time.

I took the original sensation I felt when I woke up, which was in my nervous system as a new experience, and made meaning of it right away. I was feeling "pain," which is "bad," and then referenced the past. By doing those two things, I impressed what I was feeling into my nervous system twice as deeply.

I noticed that my next thought was *I will have to go see my doctor to get him to help me with this.* Here, I time-shifted into the future, thereby impressing my experience three times more deeply into my nervous system, and I did it a fourth time when I disempowered myself from my body's ability to self-correct and heal.

Because I had been doing the work of mindfulness, I was able to watch my thoughts. I saw that my default was to time-trip into my past and plan for the future. But my angst made my situation worse because I bypassed the present moment, where the healing happens. I ceded my power to the past and future, and in doing so, I made the sensation I was feeling more intense, thereby making the body work that much harder to heal.

In this case, I noticed my thought pattern and interrupted it as soon as I began planning how soon I could see my doctor. I am not saying that doctors can't help us. Of course they can. But we can also help ourselves by not panicking, by staying present and allowing the body's wisdom to come forth. In all my time tripping, I had blocked this natural healing energy. Once I noticed what I had done, I consciously focused my thoughts on the sensation I was feeling in the present. I slowed and deepened my breathing. I sent a prayer to my Higher Power, asking for help. As I stayed quiet in the now, my attention on the breath, I felt the tightness in my neck soften and dissolve.

What a powerful lesson I learned! I was graced with a moment of clarity as I saw my thought patterns. I made a conscious adjustment by opening myself to the present moment, such a powerful ally in healing.

We are feeling creatures. In any given moment, we will feel sensations of either comfort or discomfort. The meaning we make of these sensations has a direct effect on our experience. We often have a present-moment experience but fret about how it seems like something traumatic from the past, then worry about how it will resolve in the future. This habit is one that may serve us on a survival level, but it can lead to unnecessary suffering and block our body's ability to efficiently resolve a current issue.

The Art of Passing Time

Time is our most precious commodity.

The chronic pain sufferer and addict have a common challenge: how to pass time. Ideally time is your friend, a trusted companion that is always with you. You can make time an enemy when you fight its mere existence. Because you may be uncomfortable with how you feel (and you have judged the moment to be so), you time-trip into the past or project yourself into the future, thereby missing the present moment altogether.

One of the things we learn in recovering from chronic pain and addiction is how to pass time. Let's look at it again. "Passing time" implies a fixed length of time. Yet when we are truly and fully present, the whole concept of time drops out of the equation. We are being. It's that simple. As an example, someone asked me, "How long will it take me to heal?" This is a powerful question that reveals its answer by its very form. "How long" refers to time and indicates that the person asking the question is really saying, "I don't want to be here." So, you can see the shadow that our attachment to time brings with all its implications. We can become so programmed to measure our life by time that we miss living in the present moment and all the healing that is waiting there for us.

We learn how to accept the moment with all that it brings, to fully embrace it. For me, learning the art of passing time has been a process. I made it part of my daily practice of meditation to learn to stay present. My challenge has been to stay in the present no matter what is showing up, no matter how uncomfortable, no matter how intense, no matter how much I feel fear arising within me.

I didn't say it was easy. I said it was a practice. I must keep practicing. I have noticed from doing this assignment that I have a habit of "checking out" when I have judged that things are starting to get dicey. Energetically, my default behavior is to do what I can to dissociate from my physical body, to avoid feeling what is in the moment, to distract myself from the unpleasant. That is my old habit and the old habit of many of us in recovery.

Sometimes I feel as if I must have nerves of steel to accomplish my goal of keeping myself conscious of the present moment, yet I am only flesh and blood. What I need is to come to the moment with force and fierceness, to gird myself for what I am experiencing. Yet the frequency of this energy is contracted and guarded, full of judgment and expectation. It is not the energy of allowing the experience of the moment into my being. So, you can see the challenge.

I was a smoker for decades. After I stopped smoking, I realized I needed to learn how to simply be with myself without any distraction. Smoking provided a way for me to pass time and avoid my inner experience. Instead, I had to learn to meet myself. I had to learn to settle quietly into the uncomfortable when I felt it. I had to teach my nervous system that I was safe, that I was okay, that there was no threat lurking somewhere in my periphery.

The brain of a chronic pain sufferer and addict has a strong red-alert system that is overexaggerated. Part of learning to pass time involves bringing in practices to help reset our stress response to balance. Meditation and mantra chanting are two such practices. The simple act of consciously breathing as we feel a sense of uneasiness is a potent tool for helping us pass time.

The key to healing chronic pain is to apply pain management tools daily, not only as a practice, but as a way of living. With time and daily use, I have found that those jagged edges I feel inside me have become smoother. I feel life with less urgency. The chaos and the busyness of my days in chronic pain have slowly but surely transmuted into order and the gentler movement of flow in the moment. Time slips from one moment to the next, unimpeded by my disputes and protests that I should be feeling something else, and so I am more peaceful. I have found contentment.

As I learned more about the art of passing time, I made an extraordinary discovery. Remember I mentioned all those years of time tripping into the past or the future and missing the present moment? Well, once I brought myself into the present and practiced enough to stay in it for a long enough time, I felt like I had walked right through a magical doorway. I discovered that the present moment is a vast place filled with richness I had never even imagined.

So, one of the promises of clearing chronic pain and the unhealthy habits we developed because of it is that we learn the phenomenal art of passing time. We learn how precious time truly is. We learn to flow with it instead of fight against it.

The Mind Trap: How Attention Can Sabotage Us

We can become a hostage to our beliefs, which arise from the mind. The mind can trap us and lead us in the opposite direction of where we really want to go.

For example, here's the chronic pain sufferer's typical thought pattern: *I have the pain all the time. I must control it somehow; otherwise it will hurt too much. It scares me. I feel pain no matter what I do. I am on a battlefield. I don't know when or where I'm going to get hit.*

Here's the problem: the attention is on the story of the sensation the person is feeling. It's a powerhouse of a monster story with the thoughts on the monster, not the sensation the person is feeling. There is also a lot of time tripping: "I'm in a war zone" implies that it is an eternal battle, and there's going to be a "hit," implying future tripping. Worse, the assumption that the person is going to get hit locks the cycle in even tighter.

Do you see how there is absolutely no room for healing to take place? The person may not realize it, but they have decided how their life is going to be. They have left no room at all for a different outcome for their situation; with their declaration, they have blocked their body from healing. This is my definition of self-sabotage, a mind trap if ever there was one. We become prisoners of our mind games when our attention goes here, and we become trapped.

We Can Heal from Anxiety and Panic Disorders

According to the Anxiety and Depression Association of America, anxiety disorders are the most common forms of mental illness in the United States, affecting 40 million adults age eighteen and older, or 18.1 percent of the population every year. People with anxiety disorders frequently have intense, excessive, and persistent worry and fear about everyday situations. Anxiety disorders often involve repeated episodes of sudden fear or even terror that reach a peak within minutes (panic attacks).

These feelings of anxiety and panic interfere with daily activities, are difficult to control, are out of proportion to the actual danger, and can last a long time. Sufferers may avoid places or situations to prevent these feelings. Symptoms may start during childhood or the teen years and continue into adulthood.

I suffered from anxiety and panic attacks for years in response to what seemed at the time to be chronic pain. Some of the symptoms I experienced were tension, restlessness, constant worrying, and difficulty sleeping. The doctors prescribed benzodiazepine medication to help me cope with the anxiety. However, long-term use of this class of drugs can lead to dependence and powerful withdrawal symptoms when discontinued, and it lost its effectiveness in calming my anxiety as I built up a tolerance to it. Furthermore, continual use of these drugs can end up causing more of the very problem they were prescribed for in the first place—anxiety.

Eventually I experienced more and more anxiety. This led to panic attacks, which arrived as sudden attacks of fear accompanied by a great surge of energy in my body. I felt victimized by these attacks, which seemed unpredictable, uncontrollable, alarming, and confusing because my panicky reaction was out of proportion to the level of danger around me. Most of the time I wasn't in any real danger at all. The panic attacks just seemed to come out of thin air. After experiencing several of them, I had a general sense of not feeling safe in my everyday existence.

Once I went to visit my son in Los Angeles. He was driving me to an event, and we were happily discussing where we were going. I was really happy to be with him. Then I suddenly felt that familiar surge of energy arise within me. *Oh no!* I thought. *I'm having a panic attack!* I reached into my purse, grabbed my medication, and washed it down with some water. Within a few minutes I felt the panic recede. I realized in that moment, and mentioned it to my son, that the medication hadn't even gotten a chance to get into my bloodstream before the attack subsided. Clearly, something else was at work, moderating the experience.

I did some more research on this class of medication. I was dumbfounded to discover that continued use had been found to both increase anxiety and bring on panic attacks, yet this information had not been provided with the medication, and neither the prescribing doctor nor my pharmacist had warned me about it. I decided to stop taking the medicine as soon as I could find a doctor who could help me safely withdraw from it.

I was fortunate to find a doctor to help me. I got off the medication. I learned that even though it had increased my anxiety levels, some of my behaviors were also contributing to my general anxiety disorder.

Here are some of the actions I was doing that increased my anxiety. Have you experienced any of them?

Worry and catastrophizing. I constantly worried about what was going to happen in the future. This included concern about what would happen in everyday situations, and especially after the unexpected panic attacks developed.

Fretting about past actions. I regretted things I had done in the past and had a habit of negative thinking. *I could have done it this way. I should have said it that way. If only I had done ____.*

Shallow and erratic breathing. My breathing pattern was not conducive to bringing much-needed oxygen to my body and helping to calm my nervous system. This was paramount to quieting my mind from the negative spirals of worry for the future and regret over the past.

Judging my experience. I judged the energy that I was experiencing as "bad." I labeled it anxiety or panic, which further reinforced its effect on me.

Trying to control what was happening. The more tightly I clenched my fists to control my situation, the faster the control slipped right through my fingers.

We can heal from anxiety. Here are the foundational principles to deal with it:

- The mind and body want to heal.
- You can use the ability to heal by observing Qi, or "life energy."
- You must learn to quiet your negative thoughts by using the breath and movement, such as through qigong, yoga, the Emotional Freedom Technique/Tapping, or other mindful exercises.
- Learn passive observation: you simply observe the information you are having about a direct experience.
- Stay in the present moment: life is happening here now.

- Yes, we learn from experience, and we must spend time planning for the future, but living in a constant state of worry about either is harmful.

By quieting your negative thoughts and believing in the body's ability to heal, you can let go of wanting to control your experience and allow the body's natural healing mechanism to assert itself. Let go of the past and let the future take care of itself. I had to practice these principles for a while, but my panic attacks disappeared, and the anxiety dissipated over time. Yours can, too. By incorporating these tools into your daily life, you can learn a new way to live without suffering from panic attacks or anxiety.

Healing Migraine Headaches

Migraine headaches plagued me frequently for seven years. They seemed to arrive out of thin air, made a dramatic and punishing impression, and disappeared almost as mysteriously.

My doctors and therapists tried everything they knew to help me, from chiropractic spinal adjustments to different medications. I also had help from acupuncturists, a massage therapist, a Reiki master, the practice of hatha yoga, and meditation. Each of these helped, some quickly, for a while. However, the migraines returned.

I was traumatized by these headaches, and so fearful of having them that I made sure to have my medication on me whenever I left the house. As soon as an episode started, I felt like a bomb had gone off inside my head. I immediately took my medication and waited for it to work. I just wanted the pain to go away, and I looked for any avenue that helped me get rid of it.

I implemented all the suggestions the doctors and other health care workers gave me. Even then, the migraines continued and seemed unrelenting. My life felt unpredictable, as if I were at the mercy of their attacks. I became a warrior. I fought and resisted and persevered to find a solution. Sometimes I was utterly exhausted from them. I had difficulty sleeping because I became hypervigilant. I was always either trying to prepare myself for the next headache or battling the one I was experiencing.

One day a migraine hit while I was home. I took my medication, but its effectiveness had dissipated, and I never got any pain relief. I lay in my bed, curtains drawn. Fortunately, the room was in a quiet part of the house. I lay in as comfortable a position as I could with pillows placed carefully to support my head, neck, and limbs. My head throbbed as if it might break open.

I lay still, fighting the sensations with all my might. I had tried to meditate, wanting to distract myself from what I was feeling, but to no avail. The pain persisted. Then grace came to my rescue. I heard a voice in my mind say, "Why are you doing the same thing you always do? Clearly, your strategy is not working. Why not try a contrary action?"

I wondered what "a contrary action" would be. I thought for a moment and realized how much I had been battling the headaches. I had gotten into quite a relationship with them. They were my enemy, and I treated them as such. I was judging them as something so bad that I could not tolerate their existence.

I realized that I needed to find a more neutral view. Even though it seemed scary and hopeless, I knew that the contrary action was to surrender to what I was feeling. This realization that I should stop fighting altogether was so contrary to what I normally did that it seemed a ludicrous choice. In that moment I felt the gift of desperation. What did I have to lose?

I stopped fighting. I consciously relaxed as much of my body as I could. Instead of trying to get away from the pain, I turned right into it and stared it down, gently becoming present with it. I did what I could to make what I was feeling be as neutral as possible. The pain was not my adversary, but a companion. I quietly experienced this change in my attitude and perspective. As I watched myself, the pain began to recede. Moments later, it disappeared altogether. I have never had another migraine.

What powerful lessons were here for me! I later learned that the changes I made in my behavior toward the pain were critical to helping me clear chronic pain.

Do you have this pain? Is this experience of battling with pain familiar to you? You too can find relief by shifting how you view the phenomenon of pain.

Here are the steps I took that relieved and resolved my migraine headaches:

- I worked with the health care community to find a holistic solution.
- I was open, and willing to look for a different solution.
- I listened when grace came in and suggested another approach, and trusted my intuition.
- I removed the judgment I had about the sensations I was feeling as the migraine struck.
- I stopped fighting with the migraine.
- I faced the pain instead of trying to avoid it, distract myself, or get rid of it.
- I became as neutral an actor with the migraine as I could.
- I consciously relaxed to the best of my ability.

Whatever chronic pain you are suffering from, I encourage you to try this strategy.

Healing Phantom Pain

I worked with a client who was suffering from a form of chronic pain known as phantom pain, which feels as if it's coming from a body part that has been amputated or otherwise removed. Doctors used to think that phantom pain was psychological, but it is now recognized as sensation originating in the spinal cord and brain. In this case, the source was the area where a wisdom tooth had been pulled.

I am familiar with phantom pain. I have had part of a vertebra removed, and several surgeries where bone pieces were removed from my hips for use in spinal fusions. Although this was not the same as having an entire limb amputated, the pain my client and I both experienced was diagnosed as phantom pain. This can be a particularly curious and frustrating type of pain, since the source appears to be gone. But is it really?

One of the changes we can observe in the brain of a chronic pain sufferer is how the brain interprets signals differently. Things can go a little haywire with our perceptions. We get confused because we feel something that no longer exists in the body. However, the neurological wiring to the removed part is still intact: it just needs to learn a new pathway of perception. We need to "teach it" a new way of being.

Here are things you can do to retrain the brain.

- Meditation both rests the brain so it can heal and calms the fear center in the brain.
- Be aware of your relationship to pain and shift it if necessary. Are you resisting the pain? Do you view it as an enemy, a friend, or a neutral party? Do what you can to accept the sensations you are feeling instead of resisting them.
- Stay present. It's important that you not dwell in or even reference the past regarding the pain you are feeling. It is equally important that you not worry about what your pain will be in the future.
- It's critical that you not judge what you are feeling, but instead merely experience it.
- Open yourself to the possibility of a new experience other than the pain you have felt in the past.
- Do other activities to quiet the mind, such as qigong and yoga.
- Practice every day to retrain the brain, which builds a new neural network.

Here's a powerful example of what can happen. My client with the phantom wisdom tooth pain had experienced relief and was pain-free for months. Then the pain returned. When she stopped doing her daily practice and got on with her old life, thinking she was "cured," her pain returned. As a recovering chronic pain patient, she reexperienced the pain when she no longer supported the methods that helped the brain to heal. She needed to reinstitute her daily practice to return to being pain-free.

Know that in every moment you have a choice: you can work on building your new neural network, a new highway in the brain, or you can decide to use the old neural net, thereby activating your old patterning and behaviors, and so put the old highway under reconstruction.

You can heal from chronic pain. You don't have to suffer. You just need to do the work to help the brain recover and learn anew. You need to do this practice daily.

Conclusion

Where our attention is focused and what we are doing with it has a profound effect on our pain level. It takes practice to retrain the brain to focus on the body and heal pain. In the chronic pain experience, our habit has been to ignore, distract, or numb ourselves to what we are feeling. This habit only perpetuates our suffering.

Practice making a conscious choice about where you are focusing your thoughts: either on more thought making or on the sensations arising in the body. There are times you will find yourself caught up in racing or repetitive thoughts, ruminating, or even catastrophizing. That's okay. When you notice yourself doing that, return your attention to the present moment. You may feel at some point that you are being pulled in or even down by your thoughts. Do not despair. As my friend Tiffany says, "When you're at the end of your rope, tie a knot, and climb back up."

Just stay in the present moment and feel whatever sensations in your body are coming up. Breathe and feel. You are safe, no matter what your thoughts may be saying to you.

Practice makes progress. Do your best to perfect your practice by showing up and doing it daily. You will make great progress in readjusting and healing the behaviors that kept you locked in the cycle of chronic pain. You will heal.

5

Balancing the
Negative Mind

*We have a bias toward negative thinking, which protects us
but doesn't always point us toward the best answer.*

— Elizabeth Kipp

Living with chronic pain is exhausting. It requires a lot of energy
to cope with constantly high levels of stress in the body. The
precious energy we need to handle the sensations of chronic pain
is usually accompanied by such an onslaught of negative thinking
that we can often feel as if we are bucking a current trying to
swim upstream and slowly getting pushed backward. We can
feel as if we are drowning in negativity and self-condemnation. It
is no wonder that we feel unhealthy when we are in chronic pain:
it is because we are in an unhealthy state.

Since where you focus your attention is an important part of
the chronic pain process, allowing your thoughts to stay centered
on the pain you feel feeds the pain cycle. Also part of the cycle,
negative thinking strengthens pain and draws you more deeply
into it. Careful and conscious work helps you find balance in your
thinking.

Origins of Negative Thinking

We all have negative thinking patterns, and for good reason.
Our survival instinct through the amygdala in the brain tracks
our biggest perceived threat and attends to that. Our nervous

system uses the amygdala and the vagus nerve to raise the alarm when we perceive a threat to our safety. Once we perceive a threat, these parts of the nervous system send out an alarm, setting off a chain of chemical reactions in the body that prepare us to deal with the threat.

The body releases adrenaline, noradrenaline, and cortisol as part of this fight-flight-freeze-or-faint response. The effect of these chemicals is to move blood from the center of the body to its extremities, helping us to fight or run in response to the perceived threat. The result is to see what is in front of us and get defensive, run, or shut down. We say no to keep ourselves safe from the perceived threat.

The next part of the process is when decision making begins. The left part of the prefrontal cortex activates, and we discern the level of the threat. It helps us judge the situation and reduce the level of these chemicals if the threat is less than life endangering. This activation inhibits the initial spurt of chemicals and helps us calm down. We then have the ability to match our response to the level of the threat.

Every process in the body is related to our chemistry, thoughts, and emotions. The key is that we have an alert system to keep us safe. When we are under chronic stress, our alert system and stress response get out of balance. The adrenaline in our body can take a long time to dissipate, adversely affecting our digestion, heart, and other body processes. In short, it affects our health. When the stress response is not working properly, we may respond inappropriately to something benign in the environment. We may be anxious or angry and unsure why. We have a powerful "red alert" warning system, but it needs to be in balance.

Further, we hear a warning voice in our mind that accompanies the cascade of chemical reactions occurring when we perceive a threat. This inner voice helps keep us safe. It is when we turn that voice against ourselves that we bring in self-hate and other self-destructive behaviors. We are surrounded by negativity through all the information that comes to us on any given day: the news, advertisers, other people caught in their negative thought patterns, and our own habits of negative thinking. Our brain chemistry can drive us into these patterns. It's no wonder we can feel like we are spinning in a downward spiral of negativity.

Things get even more complicated because we can become addicted to these stress hormones. People experience the surge of adrenaline and then associate the conditions and problems of life with this experience, thus reaffirming and hardening the patterning in the brain to this chemical reaction and the corresponding emotion they feel. It becomes an addiction, though they may not be conscious of it. They need the negativity to elicit the adrenaline response once more.

So these hormones of stress are highly addictive. When people link the problems of their life and use them to reaffirm their addiction to an emotion, they can become addicted to an unhealthy way of living. This is another light on the situation facing the chronic pain sufferer. The negative thinking habit itself becomes an addiction.

Under short-term stress, the body is stimulated to respond to the perceived threat and then return quickly to a balanced homeostatic state. However, in long-term stress, the body is in emergency mode indefinitely. No organism can sustain this level of stress for long. Disease sets in. Chronic pain is part of this scenario.

The Bias Toward Negative Thinking

The negative mind acts as protective energy, our early warning system and key to our survival. The positive mind helps us look for the advantage of a situation and sees the humor in it. The neutral mind does not see "good" or "bad." It speaks to us from a position of nonjudgment.

The negative mind is the first and fastest responder. Knowing this is a great advantage. When the negative mind is strong, our first response is to say no. It puts up a boundary to keep us safe. This is especially true when we find ourselves in the unknown.

"No" is a good and safe first answer, but not necessarily the best last answer. It's simply our first answer. We want to access the prefrontal cortex to navigate between the negative mind that says no and the positive mind. Ultimately, the neutral mind integrates the negative and the positive for the best response. It looks for the win-win, what's best for all. Our last answer is ideally one that reflects a healthy balance of the negative and positive minds, influenced by the neutral mind.

Please note here that we are not able to both protect and create at the same time. It's either one or the other. As long as we are in defensive mode, we only know to run, hide, freeze, or shut down in some way. This is not a space where we can access creative solutions to our dilemma. Further, the effects of the trauma that underlies chronic pain keep us from engaging with others because our patterns of connection are overridden and replaced by patterns of protection.

The Negative Bias Toward Pain

Anxiety, anger, and depression are examples of common developments in the brain that are caused by chronic pain. The cells in the brain that process emotion deteriorate faster than normal in states of anxiety and anger, so depression-like symptoms are heightened. The part of the brain involved in regulating the sleep cycle is also negatively affected. Thus, negative thinking is a result of changes the brain undergoes in the presence of chronic pain.

As organisms we have an ancient program within us about competition for resources. This is the energy frequency that says, "There's not enough" or "I better make sure there's enough for me." This trait turned in on itself manifests as "I'm not good enough." We come by it honestly: it's deeply rooted in the past.

Another aspect of this is that chronic pain sufferers can easily add to the downward spiral of negativity by allowing themselves to keep thinking negative thoughts. For example, they think about something that happened in the past that they want to change. They cannot change the past, but they also cannot stop thinking about it, because they continue to try to resolve something that is unchangeable. Such rumination is common in chronic pain sufferers.

Another adverse thinking habit is catastrophizing about future events. Again, the person cannot change the future since it hasn't yet happened, but they constantly fret about what might happen. These are thoughts of fear; they can run rampant in someone suffering from chronic pain.

We can feel like we're at the mercy of these thoughts, like we are lost in them and must fight to stay neutral, or positive and hopeful. Or we give up altogether and live in hopelessness.

Until I met Dr. Przekop, no one ever acknowledged the hopelessness I felt. I even denied it to myself. I acknowledge yours and respect you for the extraordinary journey you are on.

Please know that those suffering with this disease are doing the best they can. There is a lot of fear around living with chronic pain. We don't want to feel it, and we are afraid to try new things because we fear it might get worse. Our brain chemistry reinforces an already vulnerable state. It can seem like a perfect storm to those of us suffering from chronic pain, and the way through it often seems nebulous at best.

Chronic Pain and the Cycle of Suffering: The Dynamic

The cycle of disconnection, isolation, judgment, attachment, control, and resentment is a self-feeding and downward spiral of negativity.

Negative thinking becomes a downward spiral for the chronic pain sufferer; it leads to disconnection and isolation, judgment, attachment, control, and resentment. All types of pain, whether physical, emotional, or spiritual, are processed by the same neural connections in the brain. These connections are strengthened by repeated use and set up a negative spiral. The stress hormones produced when we experience the emotions associated with such negativity are powerfully addictive.

When healing chronic pain, we must unravel the role of the powers of control and acceptance in our experience. It is important to understand how control gets in the way. When I was in chronic pain, I, like so many others, felt that I had lost control of my body. I felt that I had no control over my healing because the pain persisted. I tried to control as much of my environment as possible, so the longer I was in pain, the more controlling my behavior became. I became obsessed with having objects in my home organized the way I wanted and got easily upset if someone moved any of them. I wanted my family members to adhere to a strict schedule for dinner and became upset when events interfered. I wanted what I wanted when I wanted it. These are classic symptoms of chronic pain sufferers and others who suffer from addictive behaviors. We find ourselves under the spell of the power of control, and acceptance is the last thing we consider.

Isolation and Disconnection

The negative cycle of suffering begins with a sense of being disconnected from our friends and family, our Higher Power, and our sense of safety in our bodies. We withdraw into ourselves as we realize that our experience is one we cannot share. Indeed, many people are distinctly uncomfortable knowing we are in pain, and we can often sense their withdrawal from us. We can feel as if we are being tested or punished, perhaps harshly, by our Higher Power. We discover that existing in our bodies is a difficult experience and may find that we have nowhere to turn for relief. We may feel trapped in our body and believe it has betrayed us. We look near and far for a solution, yet we have a great challenge in finding any respite. We look outside ourselves for the solution to our sense of disconnection, when in reality we have energetically rejected the present moment experience of our body or dissociated from it. We have left the Healing Field altogether.

Chronic pain sufferers become exceptional storytellers about their experience instead of merely experiencing it, and so miss their route to healing.

Judgment

> *The strength of your judgment is your only enemy.*
>
> — Yogi Bhajan

The negative cycle of suffering continues when we add judgment to the mix. Most of us have been raised in a culture that judges the experience of pain as "bad." The objective truth is that we feel a sensation and decide that because it is uncomfortable, it is unwanted and bad. We want to get rid of it as soon as possible. In our culture of instant gratification, the quick fix of taking a pill, although expedient at first glance, only feeds the bias of judgment. We can help unleash chronic pain's grip on us by dropping our judgment about it.

We judge the pain as bad, but it's really sensation. We are quick to reject this message from the body, call it wrong, and do whatever we can to get rid of it. Judgment is right up there with the Four Aggravations: negative thinking, resentment, procrastination, and self-doubt. The longer we feel the pain and add judgment, the higher we turn up the flame on our pain experience.

Pain is a signal that our body has been damaged. It does what it can to get us to heed its call. It will remain until the damage has fully healed. Thus, it—or, more precisely, its attenuation or disappearance—is also an indicator of healing.

I judged my pain as wrong and had taken a stand on that idea. I saw how much energy I was using to hold on to this position. It only fed into my chronic pain problem.

We judge our bodies for feeling pain. We judge them for not healing fast enough. We may judge our doctors and other health practitioners for not doing more to help us. We may even judge ourselves for not healing the way we're "supposed to" or the way someone else says we're "supposed to." We are judge and jury, and if we could, we'd also be the executioner of our pain.

The body is merely sending us a sign that we need to give it more of our attention, yet we read this signal as bad. We do our best to turn away from it. If we could just hold off on the judgment, we might realize what a miraculous healing machine the human body is. We use all sorts of energy to hold on to all the judgment around these intense sensations that we feel, thereby blocking our own healing.

All that energy could be used for healing. When we drop the energy of judgment, we lift its weight out of the equation and open the way to accelerating our healing. The body wants to heal, and it needs us as a neutral party observing our experience, not as a critic.

Attachment

This next step in the cycle of suffering is that our attachment to the pain we feel puts us in a relationship with it. When pain sent me its message, I rebelled by trying to slam the door shut—except there wasn't a door to shut. The more ways I tried to escape the pain, the more pain was waiting for me. I was codependent with it. Whenever it asserted itself, I responded in kind. My pain persisted because I remained attached to it and focused on it. All chronic pain sufferers do this.

Control

Our attempt to control our experience is the fourth factor in the cycle of suffering. We have a belief that the more we can control a situation, the safer we will be. Control becomes a kind of armor to protect us, but it creates more pain.

We identify with our story of chronic pain so much that we can't imagine living any other way. Part of that, again, is about control. We are afraid that if our life changes, it will get worse, but we also fear staying in chronic pain. We feel frustrated, and that leads to more stress and a downward spiral.

When I was in chronic pain, I felt that I had lost control of my body. I tried to control as much of my environment as possible. The longer I was in pain, the more controlling my behavior became and the more my pain grew.

Resentment

The final piece in the cycle of suffering is resentment. We have judged the sensation we feel as "bad." We want to get rid of it but cannot, so it becomes a relationship. We try to control this relationship, but that is a losing proposition. The only winner is the pain. We become resentful and angry—with the pain, with our body, and with ourselves. The outcome is more pain.

The cycle of suffering is complete. It feeds on itself, and the downward spiral into more negativity continues. Once we get to resentment, our sense of isolation deepens, and we start judging again. We become more attached to our situation and desperately try to assert control, but we fail and dive more deeply into resentment.

This is a critical dynamic for the chronic pain sufferer to understand. By seeing the behaviors that we develop when we experience chronic pain, we can begin to do the work to heal. And remember, the addictive nature of the stress hormones helps fire and wire these behaviors together so that they become more pronounced and increase our experience of negativity.

No wonder substance abuse and addiction play into this dynamic. Pain management programs with nonpharmaceutical methodologies are spread very thin as it is. Now with the rampant problem of opioid addiction, we must take the cycle of suffering into account as we develop treatment and after-treatment programs.

We have control over our attention. That is the path to finding a life out of suffering.

The difference between sensing pain and experiencing suffering is in how we handle the sensations we call "pain." The key to healing from chronic pain lies in how we react and respond to it. Do you want to resist it, fight with it, or find peace?

Use the power of acceptance. Become present. Use the neutral space of consciousness to accept what you are feeling. Put your attention on accepting what you are experiencing. Put the brakes on before you fall into judgment, rumination, and all the rest of your mental analytics. Accept the sensations you feel.

Healing Chronic Pain: Acceptance

Do not judge your healing journey—accept what it is.

Acceptance of your present moment experience is a key piece of healing chronic pain. Pain is part of life, but suffering is an option. It is critical for you to learn the difference between what you can and cannot change. What matters is your response to pain: you can choose to suffer with it, or you can choose to accept that pain is part of life.

Healing is an organic process. It is not linear, as much as you might want it to be. We can only predict the general direction toward healing. When you have an expectation of how it is going to appear or what it will look like, you limit your healing. You cannot tell your body how to heal any more than a doctor can. Get out of its way and allow the healing to happen by opening to the process.

This includes keeping your attention away from judging the pain and getting wrapped up in its story. Instead, become the neutral observer of your experience. When you release your desire to control the pain, you will find the path to healing it. It's not the road that gets you there: it's going down the road. You must walk the path to your healing by allowing the path to reveal itself to you and not judging how fast you travel down it. Your healing happens because you are traveling down the path of acceptance.

Hypervigilance and Chronic Pain

I have met many people who have developed hypervigilance with chronic pain. I developed this, too. We are always looking for the next threat, and never fully relax.

A normal stress response activates a series of physiological and emotional reactions when we perceive a threat to our survival that brings us to a full state of alertness. We are ready to act to keep ourselves safe. As we resolve the situation, our physiology and our stress response return to their normal pre-threat state.

When we experience chronic stress such as chronic pain, the normal stress response changes and can become unbalanced. The more often the stress response is activated, the harder it is to return to a normal balanced state. Hypervigilance puts the stress response on a hair trigger. We must practice mindfulness exercises to mediate this tendency toward hypervigilance, and as we reset a stress response gone awry, we retrain the nervous system to react in a healthier, balanced way.

How to Successfully Navigate the Negative Mind

Here are some tips to navigate the negative mind.

- Don't be afraid of your negative thinking. It's part of the human experience.
- There's nothing wrong with you. Your negative thinking is part of your survival.
- Be aware of what your negative thinking makes you think about yourself, others, and life.
- Know that your first response to a situation will be a negative one: "no." Ask your positive mind to reframe the original answer, then view it from the neutral mind with a nonjudgmental perspective as you seek the best solution. Of course, sometimes "no" is the right answer, and we need that boundary. We just need to make our decisions as consciously, nonreactively, and authentically as possible.
- Give yourself the space to pause before you decide.
- Remember, you are not your thoughts. You, as awareness, can watch your thoughts and not be reeled in by them.
- You need to practice *every day*. When you do, the intensity and frequency of your negative thinking habits will lessen, and their duration will shorten. You will find that you have more balance in your response to stress and you will become more resilient.

6

Genetics, Ancestral Clearing, and the Power of the Present Moment

Our ancestors live within us. They mold us into who we are.
Our ability to heal comes through this process.

— Elizabeth Kipp

Our DNA: The Unbroken Chain

An ever-so-long continuous filament reaches back more than three billion years to when the spark of life first arose on Earth. Our heartbeat alone can be traced back to the time of our ancestors' ancestors—about one billion years ago—to the common genetic information we humans share with the sea anemone. Who knows what else we share and with whom? Countless generations before us thrived, persevered, and survived cataclysms and events of epic proportion—famine, drought, disease, flood, fire, earthquakes, war, trial and error—hundreds of millions of times before you and I were born.

We are descended from survivors who passed on the message of life through the generations. Each of us is the result of so much and from so many. Our ancestors live within us, in our heartbeat, in the very marrow of our bones, in every cell of our body. They mold us into who we are. We are the culmination of all their successes. Our ability to heal comes from this process. It's part of the beautifully intricate design of the universe.

Scientists have long known that our genes carry information about our past lineage beyond eye, skin, and hair color. A relatively new field within genetics, called epigenetics, looks at the changes that arise from modification of gene expression, as opposed to *genetics*, which looks at changes caused by altering the genetic code itself.

Look to the monarch butterflies, who have lived here far longer than humans, and how their generations hold the information about their migratory path. Every fourth generation of this species makes the migration to its overwintering habitat. They find their way to their winter safe harbor even though this generation of the monarch has not previously made this journey or been there. The specific genes for migration in the monarch butterfly have not yet been identified. However, one can certainly imagine that at least some of the information about their migratory path could be found in their genetic coding.

Chronic Pain and Its Epigenetic Roots

Many studies have shown a causal correlation between emotional states and chronic pain. We hold the memories of our experiences. These include incidents we may have denied at one time because they were too painful—or we just didn't know how to deal with them. The fallout from these experiences ends up in the body, stored there until we heal the wound received from the originating event.

We also carry imprints from our parents and grandparents, and everyone back through our ancestral lineage. We have encoded within us the traits that helped our ancestors survive and their stress-related traits that weren't fatal before getting passed on to the next generation. These latter traits can carry unresolved trauma, the burdens our ancestors were unable to resolve. The burdens get passed on through our DNA; the next generation also carries those old unhealed wounds.

The Basis of Ancestral Clearing

Ancestral Clearing is a method of releasing the blocks that are sourced in our past—in this lifetime and in our ancestors' lifetimes. Unresolved burdens—such as living with a scarcity of resources; acting, for whatever reason, in ways that are selfish and to the detriment of others; not asking before taking; and being abandoned or abandoning others—are passed from one generation to the next.

Our ancestors were so busy just surviving and getting through life that they rarely if ever had an opportunity to clear the traumas and other stressful events in their lives. Since they experienced such difficult times, and because they were not able to process, clear, and resolve them, they carried this stress in their nervous system. As they reproduced, that karmic load was passed down to the next generation, and the next, and so on, down to us. We need to do what we can to acknowledge our lineage and resolve the blocks that sit squarely in the way of our being able to live in our purpose and up to our potential. These blocks can contribute to chronic pain.

How Ancestral Clearing Helps Clear Chronic Pain

The measure of the stress a human carries is termed the allostatic load. When someone experiences repeated or chronic environmental challenges, their allostatic load is a determination of the cost of their body's fluctuating or increased response by the nervous system to such stresses. It means that chronic pain sufferers carry a lot, and the load itself contributes to our pain level. How we meet stress in life is also part of the load.

We do not realize how much chronic stress weighs on us. We get used to carrying it. We are not even aware of the burden we carry from our ancestors since we have held it since birth. Sometimes we get so loaded up with these unprocessed hardships that our backs literally bend over from the weight.

Most of us, especially those of us suffering with chronic pain, move away from uncomfortable feelings. We move our attention into our thoughts, perhaps believing they are a safe place for us to focus. Given that our innate tendency is to move away from pain and toward pleasure, it is not surprising. We also tend to live our experiences in our thoughts, not our body. We make meaning of them rather than experiencing them as sensation. We will do anything to not feel the fullness of the moment. Yet the now is where the miracle of healing lies. This is the space Ancestral Clearing accesses.

When we stay in the mind, rehashing an old story or projecting how that story might unfold in the future, we are under its power. The mind will feed our story, and then the story will grow. The mind has become the master, and we give our power to it and become its servant. By dropping out of the mind and the stories it spins, we reclaim our power. To do this we must focus much more deeply into the body, where the origin of our experience lives.

When we move our attention away from the mind and into the tissues—the place we chronic pain sufferers have been trying to avoid at all costs—we find a new dynamic at play. The power of directly experiencing our life where it is centered in our body's tissues helps dissipate the tension we hold there, even to the point that we no longer feel it, thereby reducing our allostatic load.

We can hold stress from our current or past experiences, including our lineage. Let me give you an example. During World War II, my father served as a U.S. naval officer in the Pacific and my mother was a nursing assistant in the European theater. They both experienced trauma and had no way of releasing the stress they felt. Because they couldn't heal from these experiences, that stress added to their allostatic load, which they stored in their bodies. They pushed through the stress to survive. After the war, they met, fell in love, married, and had my brother and me.

They passed the tension from their experiences of the war on to us. My brother and I did not have the memory of these events, but we felt them as tension in our nervous system. Because I was born holding this energy, I never realized I was carrying it until I experienced Ancestral Clearing and literally "cleared" it out of my nervous system.

An Example of an Energetic Frequency

It never occurred to me that forgiveness would be such a key player in releasing the weight of my allostatic load and recovering from chronic pain. I was simply used to dealing with life the only way I knew: things happened, I experienced them, they felt uncomfortable. I had no clue what to do with all that discomfort, so I did what I thought everyone around me did: I pretended it wasn't there and distracted myself from feeling it. I even numbed it. I never healed the wounds that were created when I experienced adversity, and built up anger about it. It never crossed my mind that this was something forgiveness could help remedy.

The constant state of pain fed discouragement, yet I needed some ray of hope. The longer I felt pain, the more frustrated I became. Afraid to make any change, I could not release past mistakes and disappointments. I worried constantly about the future. Fear, disappointment, anger, and sadness were all ingredients that fueled my chronic pain.

Notice that this describes a certain energy frequency, one of fear, lack, scarcity, time tripping, and negative thinking. (See Chapters 4 and 5.) This energy has a momentum, one we may have come into this life with from our parents and ancestors that is also the driving force of the subconscious programming affecting our behaviors because of events in this lifetime. The good news is that we can shift this frequency.

We Begin with Awareness

In my case, I first had to face my fear. I made the decision that enough was enough, and I confronted my pain—all of it. I encourage you to take this step, too. Until we face our fears, we never know our capacity for courage. That is the beginning point of healing our pain.

Let me take you to a different energetic frequency, from one of fear and worry to one of hope and courage. While I spent much of my time in the energy of fear, tucked down deep inside of me was the insistent calling of my inner knowing, my soul. I just had a difficult time hearing it through all the chaos of chronic pain and the constant state of fear that accompanied it.

I discovered Ancestral Clearing through the pioneering efforts of Howard Wills and John Newton. John brought this work to Dr. Przekop's Pain Management Program. This modality helped me find freedom and healing from chronic pain.

My Experience with Ancestral Clearing and Forgiveness

Let me give you a specific example of some of the magic packed within Ancestral Clearing work:

The word *forgive* has its origins in "to forgo or give up."

If I intellectually forgive someone but do not remove the emotional charge from the event I'm forgiving around, then I have not fully forgiven. I'm *not* saying I'm condoning the behavior I am forgiving: I'm saying I'm *fully* forgiving. I might say, "I forgive my mother, but I'll never forget what she did to me." By not forgetting, I am always going to protect myself from being hurt like that again and I am unwilling to let the incident go altogether. That is *not* true and full forgiveness.

So, if I'm having a challenging time truly forgiving my mother, what do I do? Where do I turn? I turn to a power greater than myself to help me take this difficult step. Clearly, I have not found a way to let it go by myself. My being stuck here is not good for my mother either.

I ask, "Higher Power, all that You are, help me forgive my mother, no matter what she did. Help her to forgive me, and help us to forgive ourselves, completely and totally. Please and thank You." Yes, I cried when I said this. With those tears, I felt a release in my body. The emotional charge that had been built up inside my body, literally in my tissues, dissipated. Because I asked for help, my Higher Power helped me transcend this block of resentment toward my mother. I was graced with a liberating release and felt humility and gratitude. Without true forgiveness I would not be addressing the core of the problem and it would reemerge.

And so it can be for us all. We take responsibility for our part in a situation. This is healing. We use forgiveness in prayer as a vehicle by which to release emotional energy. The use of prayer and its connection to Higher Power leads us to our own liberation through the humble and grateful act of forgiveness itself. When I did this, I felt my physical pain recede into swirls of energy that flowed through and ultimately out of my body. The pressured tension of pent-up emotional pain was released in a cascade of tears and resulted in a profound inner release. I witnessed this same healing in other patients in the Pain Management Program as they did this practice.

Ancestral Clearing: The Process

The practice of Ancestral Clearing involves awareness, remembering our connection to the Higher Power of our understanding, forgiveness, gratitude, and humility.

The brain can heal only in the present. It does not exist in the past or the future. We must be in the present or we will suffer. If we are in the habit of slipping into the past or stressing about the future, we miss the present altogether. Ancestral Clearing brings us right into the present moment where the healing takes place. We become aware of the sensations we feel when we think about the things we want to forgive.

The next step in the Ancestral Clearing practice is being willing to forgive, to let go. We can get attached to our resentments, get into a relationship with them, and get used to them being around. To use the tool of forgiveness to help heal chronic pain, we must first be willing to give up our attachments to these negatives in our life, however familiar and even comfortable we have become with them.

We next humbly ask for help from a Higher Power to help us forgive. My experience with this work is that you don't need to believe in a Higher Power. The only requirement to getting this kind of help is to want the help. We forgive the pain, and we forgive the body for hurting all the time. We forgive missing life because we were in pain. We forgive others for judging us and our pain. We forgive ourselves for judging others and ourselves. We forgive others for the hurts we have received. We forgive the loneliness we feel in our experience of chronic pain. We forgive all that we can in the moment. We allow ourselves to feel what comes up for us as sensation as we reference and forgive the hurts, and because we are feeling the sensations in the present, the body can release them.

Here's the thing about forgiving the burden we carry. We never know how heavy the burden is until we have done the work of forgiving. We carried it for so long that we got used to its weight. Or we thought we did. The body knew better. It groaned and complained under the weight until it finally expressed itself as chronic pain. When we practice forgiveness, we release the load of the unresolved hurts we experienced. With that energy released, we feel lighter, because we have literally lightened the burden and healed the damage done from the allostatic load we carried.

Finally, we give thanks to our Higher Power for the release of the weight and tension from the old hurt we were carrying.

I found so much relief from forgiveness and Ancestral Clearing that I became a practitioner of the work. Many others have found peace and ease in their lives through the healing of Ancestral Clearing. You can, too. This work is complementary to and supportive of the work of doctors, therapists, and other health care professionals.

Ultimately, forgiveness is a quiet, private journey one takes deep down, where we feel our wounds the most, and in that place where we feel the loving energy of the Infinite. It's not on the outside, not a spiritual bypass, spoken with the pretense of proving we're bigger or more evolved, or more kind or loving. It is a personal walk to the core of our being where we forgive the source of our hurts and grow our capacity for courage to let them go and live free from their burden. It is a simple yet potent tool to help clear chronic pain.

The Power of the Present Moment

The power of being in the present moment cannot be overstated, especially when it comes to healing. The present *is* the place of transformation. The past cannot be changed, and the future has yet to occur, so when else would healing take place? Yet we often miss seeing this space for the power broker it is in our life.

If we bring the story of our past into the present, we have biased our experience. Whatever shows up in the present will be colored by this story. For instance, if I am resentful toward someone and my attention stays on that situation as I sit in the present, then I carry my bitterness into the moment. I might even find that my further attention to it drives it more deeply into my experience.

On the other hand, when I access the moment as a mere witness without judgment, I might notice that resentment comes into my field of consciousness. In this space, I notice what sensations are arising in my body as the thought comes. I can add a forgiveness prayer for myself and all my ancestors for any time anyone held on to a resentment. I humbly and gratefully ask my Higher Power to please help us all forgive each other for resentments. Here I use the power of presence and Higher Power energy to clear the charge or tension I was feeling about the resentment as I noticed it show up.

That is what healing looks like.

That is the power of the present moment.

There is something profound and mysterious about becoming a blank slate, when our only participation in the present is in observing what is arising in our awareness. Here there is no effort, only openness. We bring an open heart and a willing mind and focus into the present, meeting life on life's terms. We accept whatever is here. We feel the flow of energy. We come without an agenda, only openness. The present moment is always arising anew. In this way it is a mystery to us, and we are living the Mystery by being it.

The Pause and Its Importance in Healing Chronic Pain

We can be so caught up in our thoughts that it's as if we are on an endlessly spinning hamster wheel. If we look at it from the perspective of physics, we can say that this spinning has its own momentum. To get off the hamster wheel, we must change its momentum.

Enter the pause. All we need to do is pause for a moment to change the momentum of our spinning thoughts completely. The pause is a sumptuous and sacred space of creativity.

Look to the cell as an example. When a cell divides, whether through mitosis or meiosis, the stage (resting or interphase) just before that moment of creativity is the pause. It is a place of stillness and fundamental reorganization. From this resting phase—this pause—is born the next phase of creating something new.

Here is how I see the part the pause plays in the life of the addict and chronic pain sufferer.

When we are caught up in our thoughts, it is as if we are lost in a great deluge or avalanche. The momentum is that powerful. We can be so lost in it that we don't even realize we are lost.

Imagine what would have to happen to pause a waterfall or an avalanche. The power it would take to do that is the same kind of power it takes to stop the avalanche of our thoughts. That there is a way to disengage from the cascade of our thoughts is a miracle when viewed from this perspective. Yet that is how powerful the pause is.

I understand that you might question how one might pause the flow of a waterfall, or how an avalanche can slow down. We base our predictions on what we have known to be true in our past. But here's the thing: this is the limited thinking we are locked into when we suffer with chronic pain. I know: I lived it.

I wanted to think outside the box. I knew that kind of thinking was out there somewhere, but I just couldn't access it. I had no empirical evidence in my past that would point me to a life other than the one I was living. I was caught in my own version of the endlessly spinning thoughts of the typical addict and chronic pain sufferer.

It was an extraordinary and powerful occasion for me when I was shown a new possibility, embraced it, and felt the shift in my experience as the pain dissolved back into the void from which it had arisen. I found it hard to believe, yet it was indeed happening. It was so momentous that as I look back on it, it seems as if someone came along and turned off the flow of the waterfall of pain rushing inside me. It's as though the avalanche of chaos that was my life suddenly switched from careening downhill to climbing steadily back up the mountain of wellness.

Amid all this abrupt change in the direction of my health was the pause—the pause, when all things as I knew them stopped for one moment as I considered that there might be another way to live, even if I wasn't exactly sure what it was. A new possibility arose from that place of pause. It was the turning point for me, the pivot point around which all else rotated. It was the place from which, moving forward, my choices made all the difference.

The pause is a sacred place for many reasons. As in the example of the cell, it is that space from which creativity arises. For the addict, it can be the bottom from which all else springs. It is the place where at last we say, "Enough! There must be another way." We are at the brink, and we come face-to-face with ourselves. It is a place of raw, stark, and rich honesty.

To heal, you need to be willing to sit in the uncomfortable. It is all part of the miraculous healing power of the body. You are releasing toxic stuff. It's going to feel strange and not exactly blissful. You can do this while sitting with a therapist. You can sit with your Higher Power. You can sit with your Self. Remember: you are not your body; your body is in you. So, feel and release. Do not judge what you are feeling; just feel it. Your body will take care of whatever this uncomfortable thing is in the most magnificent way. That is the power the pause gives us.

For the chronic pain sufferer, the pause is also where we finally come to a place where we are no longer terrified of our pain. In the pause, we turn and face our pain, if only for a millisecond. We meet it. And in this pause, we switch from ceding our power to the pain to taking our power back. We move from victimhood to empowerment. It is the springboard from which we rise.

A lot of energy exists in this moment of pause around which all other momentum revolves. It is the turning point. It is the point of healing. It is from this pause that we can step into the power of presence and its miraculous healing potential.

Challenges in Chronic Pain Recovery

Understand that the person who has lived in the suffering of chronic pain has become an expert, an Olympic-level athlete, at holding on. We have a program running deep in us that is sending the message and powerful belief that "I'm not safe—ever." We believe this story. We buy into this story hook, line, and sinker because hypervigilance has become part of our life.

Here's the dilemma. We have been holding on to our defenses, holding ourselves stiff and armored up, guarding our flanks and our hearts for so long that we forget where the muscles are that are doing all the holding, armoring, and guarding. Try to imagine what it's like to feel the sweet warmth of the sun on your skin after you have been in the cold dark for so long that you'd forgotten the sun altogether.

The chronic pain sufferer is closed and not likely to take the risk of opening themselves for fear of that opening going wrong. The chronic pain sufferer dreads that the opening may backfire and that they will end up shutting down and collapsing altogether. This fear is like an all-points fire alarm going off all the time.

In recovery, the medications and the old lifestyle have been taken away. The person's belief system is also being turned upside down. This is some eye-opening, daring territory. The trade-off, of course, is the promise of recovery, of healing. Going from closed down in defense mode as a chronic pain sufferer to cracking that well-worn armor wide open is an epic journey!

The wonder of learning to be present, practicing meditation, quieting the mind, and adding the Ancestral Clearing work to the mix is that these modalities together provide a powerfully healthy shake-up to this entire system. This work cracks the hard shell of protection of the chronic pain sufferer's world. These tools clear the decks for us so that we can find those long-lost muscles that have been holding us back and let them go at last. We switch the nervous system from being in defense mode, where only protection is possible, to relaxation, and so switch into the creative powers that live in it. We literally change our body chemistry in this process and so heal the detrimental changes chronic pain brought to us.

We learn to let the past go, maybe little by little, but surely. We learn to rest in the present and not borrow trouble by imagining that our next moment will be a catastrophe. We learn to begin to trust that our body really does have the power to heal, because we begin to feel better.

Further, when we are in early recovery, we find ourselves suddenly lit up with sensation, which is a new experience for us. We also feel our emotions more vividly and must learn to deal with that bias to the negative mind. Learning to be present, quieting the mind, clearing our past—these are the core tools that will help us heal.

When we use these tools, we place ourselves directly on a path to healing. We shift from desperately and ineffectively trying to control our chronic pain to being able to control our healing. Note what a shift that represents: from resigning ourselves to the belief that we are going to hurt and trying to manage living like that to implementing a plan to change our life so that we heal from the pain.

(7)

The Twelve Steps
of Chronic Pain

*Surrender can help the chronic pain sufferer reset the stress
response, calm the mind, and find inner peace.*

— Elizabeth Kipp

Surrendering the Fight with Pain

Chronic pain sufferers are some of the most hope-filled people in the world. But they can descend into hopelessness. Our issues with control dovetail here. When viewed from the point of view of surrender, the twelve steps of chronic pain can help chronic pain sufferers in recovery regain their footing by helping to reset the stress response, calm the mind, and find inner peace and contentment.

Like all addicts, chronic pain sufferers are control freaks. We take our compulsion for control to the next level.

Here's how this works: We feel enough sensation to be uncomfortable in our skin. We cannot escape it, though we do what we can to not feel all the sensory signals firing inside us. We try in every way possible to control the situation.

Our body is doing its best to send a signal warning us to change what we are doing. With chronic pain, the signal persists, beyond pain medication and whatever behaviors that are contributing to our predicament. Our doctors often know nothing more than to give us medication, but even though we use what we think will mediate or calm the signals, we continue to feel the sensations.

We decide to continue the hunt for another way to control our experience: the opposite of accepting what we are feeling. The metaphor I use here is standing at the bottom of Niagara Falls and pushing up on the water, trying to make it stop flowing. See how hopeless that is?

Here is the amazing paradox of a chronic pain sufferer: desperate to control our situation, we come up against an impenetrable wall, yet we continue. This is hope in the face of all odds. It is also classic human behavior: doing the same thing over and over while hoping for a different outcome. This hopefulness, despite a track record of failure, keeps us coming back to try and try again.

Our brains change so much from the experience of chronic pain that we become utterly rattled. We fight the sensations, but ultimately, we end up fighting ourselves. The concept of surrender, to the pain or anything else, is foreign to us. It sure was for me.

Chronic pain sufferers get caught in a war with intense sensation in a body we cannot escape. The miracle is that we continue to seek a solution. In my case, I continued for years, intuitively feeling that solution just beyond my reach.

At some point we reach a sacred bottom. We have had enough pain and enough of struggling with the pain. We're done and we know it. Surrendering to the pain becomes our only option. It is in this surrender point that we turn into our powerful Healing Field, where the miracle begins anew in a heretofore unimaginable form.

Where we were once trying to push the water of Niagara Falls back up, we are now letting go of the fight. In doing so, we enter the flow of the water and become one with it. We no longer fight—we flow. We get out of the way and empower the body to assert its awesome healing powers.

The Miracle of Surrender

In active addiction, I knew surrender was inevitable: it was only a matter of time and circumstances. The possibility of any kind of recovery seemed highly questionable to me, and any shot at it had all but faded to the barest glow on the edge of my inner horizon. I was so lost in the chaos of chronic pain and addiction that I could not even conceive that recovery was possible. The gifts of recovery are in many ways completely unexplainable to those who have not experienced such spiritual metamorphosis themselves.

I experienced my recovery as surrender on many levels. I surrendered my willfulness to exert control at all costs. I surrendered my conviction that I was right. I surrendered my perspective. I surrendered my hopelessness. I surrendered my insanity. I surrendered to the pain. I surrendered my selfishness. I bowed such a bow I will never forget. I laid it all down at the feet of whatever that unknowable but ever-present Higher Power was. And in the process I was released from the isolation I had known for so long and gained back the connection to my Self, the world, and my Higher Power. I experienced a profound spiritual awakening.

The Twelve Steps of Chronic Pain

Here are the twelve steps of chronic pain. I offer them as a bow, surrendering all and gaining everything, all the gifts of recovery, in return.

Step 1. I bow to how unmanageable my life has become.
Step 2. I bow to the idea that there is a Power greater than me.
Step 3. I bow to the concept that such a Power can help me find my way out of the chaos. I bow to this Higher Power, and I keep bowing.
Step 4. I bow to all the different and seemingly disparate parts of myself.

Step 5. I bow to my Higher Power and find faith in another person and in myself, which helps me embrace all of who I am.

Step 6. I bow and open myself to my Higher Power and ask to change and grow.

Step 7. I bow to all those I have harmed in any way and become willing to make amends.

Step 8. I bow to my trespasses and make amends where I can.

Step 9. I bow to the truth in my daily actions and course correct every night, admitting my mistakes.

Step 10. I bow and bow again to my Higher Power and ask for guidance and the power to act on such guidance.

Step 11. I bow, and in the light of the bow, hold it for those seeking a way out of the darkness.

Step 12. I bow and pray that I will find the power and the wisdom to keep bowing.

The twelve steps used for Alcoholics Anonymous, Narcotics Anonymous, Codependency Anonymous, and many other twelve-step programs, including Chronic Pain Anonymous, are useful as part of the healing process. Here are a few notes about how to apply the principles outlined in this book to the twelve steps.

The main issue with someone dealing with chronic pain is control. Because we perceive chronic pain as pervasive and overwhelming, we try desperately to control our lives wherever we can. Part of healing this destructive pattern is learning to renounce our insistence on having control. We find that our perspective on the power structure readjusts. We realize who is really in charge: our Higher Power, not us. Knowing this, we can finally relax that tension we have been holding for so long. These actions help us unleash our healing power. These twelve steps underline the action of bowing, of relinquishing our power to a power greater and more loving than ourselves, and in the process, help lead us to a spiritual awakening.

Take note in the section below that the word *we* is in all these steps. We are no longer isolated. We seek out others who are working to recover, and enlist their help. We do this work in a group setting, at minimum with a sponsor who can help guide us through the process.

These twelve steps are written as personal action steps. Remember, I see the terms *chronic pain sufferer* and *addict* interchangeably.

Step 1: We admit we are powerless over our addiction, that our lives have become unmanageable.

In this step, we embrace a sacred moment. We realize we have come to the brink. We can take no more. We realize we have ceded our power to the pain, our habit of engaging it, our addiction to it, our desire to control. We admit our lives have become unmanageable. Step 1 is a place of the bow, the sweet relief of humility. It is the first step in regaining our power. We get honest with ourselves and bow to our situation and ourselves. We shift from hiding from ourselves to facing ourselves with the truth about our situation.

In Step 1, we bow in surrender and accept where we are.

Step 2: We come to believe that a Power greater than ourselves can restore us to sanity.

In Step 2, we finally realize that our way of thinking has brought us to this point. We see that our way of doing things has not led to health. The root word for sanity is *sanus*, meaning "healthy." We see that our behaviors have fed our suffering. In this way, we are insane. Clearly, we were unable to find a healthy way to live by ourselves.

We know from our honest look at ourselves in Step 1 that we are utterly overwhelmed. In Step 2 we look to a Power that is even greater than our addiction and our suffering.

In Step 1, we came to the brink. We came to the pause. *Now in Step 2, we take a leap. And as we leap, we are bowing once again in humility. We change the direction of our previous momentum.*

Step 3: We make a decision to turn our will and our lives over to the care of a Higher Power greater and more loving than us.

In Step 3, we bow once more to a Higher Power of our understanding who is greater and more loving than ourselves. Before, we tried to control our pain and our lives only to find they became more uncontrollable. We felt the grip of chronic pain tighten and intensify. We repeated this strategy, never succeeded, and sank more deeply into the abyss of suffering.

We had lived in isolation before and tried to work everything out by ourselves. We were so overwhelmed by our pain that we turned away from friends, family, and ourselves. Our disconnection was complete and terrifying, and we coped by trying to control everything we could.

In Step 3 we turn everything over to our Higher Power. This is a place of humility and great relief as we realize we can enlist a Higher Power to act as our guide.

In Step 3, we turn willfulness into willingness.

Step 4: We make a fearless and moral inventory of ourselves.

Step 4 invites us to look at the underpinnings of our pain. We do not have to relive old traumas. Instead, Step 4 is a place of deep listening. It's a further dive into Step 1, immersing ourselves even more deeply into the truth of our past. We are not dwelling here, but we remain long enough to give voice to those parts of ourselves we have ignored or tried so desperately to silence for so long.

We look at our liabilities and our assets regarding our character and our actions. For some of us, this may be the first time we have done this.

We also bring self-compassion. Before doing any step work, my sponsors and I have always started with a prayer to our Higher Power. This is one more place to bow and turn our will over to willingness. In the prayer, we ask for courage and compassion as we work Step 4.

As chronic pain sufferers, we have been filled with fear of our pain. With the help of our Higher Power, we take the reins of power back. In our honest assessment, by listing what we are so upset about, we realize how much resentment and anger we have built up about our pain and whatever we believe caused it. We may be angry with the body, others, our Higher Power, or ourselves.

We examine the fear that lies beneath the surface of our anger. The more we fought our pain, the harder we tried to get rid of it, and the bigger it, and our fear of it, grew. We see this conundrum and the prison we made for ourselves.

Please note that Step 4 is a key place to practice self-compassion. We can look back at what happened and marvel that we stuck with things and survived to this moment. We can thank ourselves and our Higher Power. This is another step where we bow.

In Step 4, we shift from fearful to fearless. I am not saying that we are no longer afraid of pain. I am saying that we are no longer afraid of facing ourselves, our secrets, and our shame.

We keep secrets out of fear of others' reactions, fear of being the object of ridicule, fear of being rejected, punished, and even persecuted. We keep secrets out of shame. We close to others and close to ourselves. We close our hearts. We hide things so deeply that sometimes we even forget they are there. Yet we feel them. Their impact never goes away. They begin to fester and grow.

Shame feeds addiction. So, as recovering addicts, we become brave shame hunters. We do what we can to seek it out and shine a bright, disinfecting light on it. No longer will it hide and eat away at our very foundation. When we go after our shame, we get a good handle on preventing relapse and open ourselves even more widely to healing.

In Step 4, we shift from living in fear to becoming fearless.

Step 5: We admit to our Higher Power, to ourselves, and another human being the exact nature of our wrongs.

Step 5 helps us further solidify our work in Step 4 by sharing all the work we did in the prior step with another person, our sponsor. The secrets we've hidden away for so long are not only out to ourselves, but to the world through that person. Speaking these newly unearthed truths acts as a kind of rich compost that helps our healing grow even deeper.

We have brought ourselves further and further out of isolation with each step. Step 5 cements our commitment to getting truthful with ourselves by declaring our truths to someone else. I see it as a step where we literally declare our commitment to our healing.

It can be in a moment of such power that our healing takes on a new dimension. We are more self-aware, and we have decided to embrace who we have found in ourselves.

In Step 5, we become even more fearless.

Step 6: We are entirely ready to have the Higher Power of our understanding remove all these unhealthy behaviors.

For me, this step is where the rubber meets the road. Let me explain.

The first time I read Step 6, I read it as if it said, "We are entirely ready, and now God will remove all these unhealthy behaviors." That is not quite what it says. My sponsor lovingly pointed this out to me when I asked her, "How can my Higher Power take away all of my unhealthy behaviors?" This step says that we are now *ready and willing* to do the work, not that it will be taken away.

Our Higher Power is there for us, of course. However, the work is done by both of us. It is a co-creative process.

After writing out our personal inventory and sharing it with our Higher Power and another person, we get down to work of a different kind in Step 6. We are ready to release the burdens we have been carrying for so long. The action here is in bowing and asking our Higher Power to help us let go and then pray in stillness, showing that we are ready to purge and purify ourselves.

In Step 6, we double down on our willingness from Step 3. We bow to our Higher Power, open ourselves, and ask to change and grow.

Step 7: We humbly ask our Higher Power to remove our shortcomings.

When I read Step 7 the first time, I thought my Higher Power was going to remove my shortcomings. That's not the way it works. In this step, we are ready for our assignment. So, we *ask* our Higher Power to remove all our unhealthy behaviors.

For example, I have had an incredible challenge with patience. First, I realize my impatience is an unhealthy behavior. Then, I humbly ask my Higher Power to help remove my impatience. The juice and the magic of Step 7 come next. I go on living my life, and the next thing I know, I am dealing with a situation that tries my patience. I find myself face-to-face with whatever it is that irks me. *This* is my Higher Power in action. I ask for help from the Boss, and lo and behold, I receive it. Maybe not the way I want it, but my request is granted. My Higher Power has a sense of humor, too. I will continue to be presented with the lesson of patience until I learn it. Such is the power of Step 7.

In Step 7, we bow and open ourselves to our Higher Power, and ask to change and grow. **We get to work on ourselves, removing unhealthy behaviors and building our integrity.**

Step 8: We make a list of all persons we have harmed and become willing to make amends to them all.

In Step 8, once again, we bow. Our personal inventory from Step 4 lists the resentments we have and the times when we have harmed other people. In Step 8, we list the people we harmed. We build our willingness once more. Bowing to our Higher Power for guidance, we open ourselves and become willing to make amends. We bow to those we have wronged, including ourselves. Self-compassion and self-forgiveness are at the core of Step 8. I remember feeling a deep measure of peace as I did the work for this step. It was a relief to know that it was possible for me to make such amends.

In Step 8, we bow to all those we have harmed in any way and become willing to make amends.

Step 9: We make direct amends to such people wherever possible, except when to do so would injure them or others.

In this step, we further our work of purifying ourselves by coming clean to people we have wronged. With the help of our Higher Power and all the work done in the previous steps, we can face those we have injured in some way. We make an adjustment in our relationships here, including our relationship with ourselves. *Amend* means "to adjust or rework." We are righting the ship, so to speak, and clearing the decks. We go to the people we have hurt and admit our wrongdoings.

This step is one of liberation, because doing it means we have been honest and cleaned up our past. Through our actions, we have released the pent-up energies of guilt and shame around our past behaviors and come clean with those against whom we trespassed. When we bow earnestly to our Higher Power, our transgressions, and those we have harmed, we rise above our circumstances.

In Step 9, we bow to our trespasses and make amends where we can, and in the process, we are liberated.

Step 10: We continue to take personal inventory, and when we are wrong, we promptly admit it.

Here in Step 10, we once again take responsibility for our actions. We take the lessons we learned in the previous steps and apply them in all our actions. Living in integrity becomes a lifestyle to which we aspire. We work this step on a regular basis so that it becomes part of our nature.

This step helps us live in the moment and not allow ourselves to carry resentments. We own our mistakes. We take responsibility for our lives. We replace playing the victim with living a role of empowerment.

In Step 10, we bow to the truth in our daily actions and course correct every night, admitting our mistakes. We stay in integrity with ourselves.

Step 11: We seek through prayer and meditation to improve our conscious contact with our Higher Power as we understand it, praying only for our Higher Power's knowledge of its will for us and the power to carry that out.

Because of the work we did in the previous steps, in Step 11 we can strive toward including our conscious contact with the Higher Power of our understanding in everything we do. This is an important step, because we are no longer living our life from a place of trying to control everything. Instead, we look to our Higher Power for guidance. Thy will, not my will, be done. This step is where the rubber meets the road once more. The action here is to bow, ask, listen, and act once we hear divine guidance.

In Step 11, we bow and bow again to our Higher Power, and ask for guidance and the power to act on such guidance.

Step 12: Having had a spiritual awakening as a result of these steps, we try to carry this message to other addicts and to practice these principles in all our affairs.

We have found our way through the darkness of chronic pain and addiction. Now we have the opportunity, honor, and responsibility to pass the torch forward. We are now the light in the darkness for those who still suffer.

We work this step in a few ways.

We live by example. We build on all the other steps, for they culminate here in Step 12. By living in humility with the guidance of our Higher Power, we live the example of what the steps outline for us.

We live by being of service to others. We work in community, within a twelve-step fellowship, or perhaps in an institutional setting, and carry the message of recovery. This is not an evangelistic or promotional pursuit, but one in which our behavior becomes attractive to others. Occasions will present themselves to us to help others find their way through the suffering of chronic pain and addiction.

In Step 12, we bow, and in the light of the bow, hold it for those seeking a way out of the darkness. We bow and pray that we will find the power and wisdom to keep bowing.

There is much discussion about "power" in recovery, in the literature, and in the steps. I have wrestled with this. I have been in discussion with a few people about "powerlessness" versus "getting our power back." It has been an ongoing conversation since 2013. These words get tossed around and can be really confusing.

For instance, if we admit we are powerless over our addiction, how can we even speak of "regaining our power"? And, if we are "turning it [read, our power] over" to our Higher Power, then we have no power at all, because we just turned it over, right? See how confusing that sounds?

Here's what really makes sense to me, now that I've turned the entire matter over to my Higher Power and quietly listened for a response. We call back our inherent power and empower ourselves through this act of surrender.

In our addiction, we have lost ourselves and live as this weird shadow of who we are. We are splintered into aberrant versions of ourselves. We have lost track of our wholeness and our health on every level. When we do the twelve steps and other work in recovery, we turn our power over to our Higher Power as the ultimate authority. With its help and our honesty, willingness, and openness, we reclaim or call back those parts of ourselves from addiction.

We may be powerless over our addiction, but with the help of a Higher Power, we reconnect to those parts of us that splintered away. We incorporate that weird shadow back into ourselves, and through the transformational ability of step work, we become whole and healthy again. The power, therefore, is in our becoming whole and healthy.

It is not so much about "power" versus "powerlessness" as it is about the integration of ourselves with the direction of our Higher Power. We get the power structure straight and reclaim our lost selves.

The twelve steps create a structure for us to actively practice how to live beyond selfishness and victimhood. They teach us how to release the fierce grip of control we felt we needed as addicts. We have found a place beyond hopelessness. We are caught by our Higher Power and realize we are held and will not be dropped. When we bow, we rise out of the victimhood of our circumstances and into empowerment. We find sweet relief. We find an honesty we had hoped for but didn't realize was possible. We discover that we are not alone. We find joy and purpose in service to others. We find a new way to live. We find liberation. And in the process, we find ourselves.

Mindfulness
and the Breath

*The value of a meditation practice to a chronic pain
sufferer is that it provides a powerful and effective
technique for unhooking us from the pain. In this, it is an
indispensable healing tool.*

— Elizabeth Kipp

We are born on an inhale. We die on an exhale. Our breath
defines and moderates our entire existence. The quality of
our breath determines the quality of our lives. This is knowledge
the ancient yogis knew well; so did every doctor I ever knew
who was worth their salt. We can hold the breath in reaction
or breathe consciously with ease and purpose. Our use of the
breath affects how we feel and our overall health.

Cracking the Code to Chronic Pain: Meditation

We can get hooked in our pain.

Eckhart Tolle calls it the pain body: our accumulation of
unresolved traumas and hurts that remain locked in our cells. It's
even more than that, I think.

We get in relationship with our pain. We give our power away
to it. We get all tangled up in it, as if we are caught up in a spider's
web. We fight the pain. We try to make it go away. We try to hide
from it. We do not want to accept it for what it is. So long as we
remain wrapped up in dealing with our pain, it sits on our throne
and we are its servant.

Learn to observe the pain instead of being captured and enveloped by it. Experience yourself watching the pain and watching yourself in it. Realize you are not your pain. This is a critical tipping point that begins to direct the momentum away from suffering. It permanently tears through and penetrates the great mass built up in the pain body.

In meditation you learn to become the watcher.

Meditation teaches you that you no longer have to do anything at all: you no longer have to fight the pain, no longer have to try to make the pain do this or that. You sit and watch yourself. Once you as the watcher become separated from it, the fierce grip that pain has on you will begin to loosen and fall away. You need only continue to practice your meditation in earnest. In the end, in choosing to no longer give your power away to it, you yourself are the one who releases the grip of pain.

Our breath has its origins in the sea and in single-celled organisms. Everything that is alive has respiration as its foundation. We all know how to breathe. We do so unconsciously, and we are blessed to have this ability. Yet there is great power in our learning to make the breath a conscious act. When we are calm, even unconsciously we breathe more deeply and slowly than we do when we are stressed. As we feel life's pressures, we tend to shorten and even hold our breath altogether, especially when we are startled or feel threatened.

The heartbeat follows the breath. As we experience stress, our breath quickens and becomes shallower. Our heartbeat follows suit, speeding up and even becoming more erratic than regular. We feel this as increased chaos and discomfort in the body and wonder, *What happened?* When we bring consciousness to our breathing, we can deeply calm ourselves and bring the heartbeat back to its normal rhythm.

Meditation with the breath helps bring peace into your life when you feel tension and chaos. You have a choice in how you respond to the stresses and strains that can erupt in your life. It is one way to calm yourself and live more from a place of choosing to respond instead of reacting to events.

The mind is a giant recording machine. All our experiences, beliefs, and habits are recorded in the subconscious mind. About 90 percent of the mind is subconscious and 10 percent is conscious, so you can imagine how great an effect the 90 percent has on our decision making.

When we're talking about renewal of the mind, we're talking about healing through presence and repatterning unhealthy behaviors. When you apply presence, you begin to clean the lens of perception and see with different eyes. This starts to repattern the brain. Those deep patterns that get created in the subconscious mind, that are driving us, start to shift. And when the inner patterns of the mind start to shift, the outer reality starts to shift. In this process of renewal, inside and outside, our healing unfolds.

The most powerful way to initiate such healing is to meditate.

What Meditation Looks Like

When you are in meditation, you take the role of the witness. Observe what you are experiencing in your body and thoughts and what's happening in the world around you. Continue noticing what is in your awareness. Remain in this place of being the observer to yourself.

You may be focusing on the breath, a mantra, or just the quiet in the moment. Notice if you are being still or are being triggered and unsettled by what is happening within or around you. There is no judgment here, just noticing and awareness. This is presence.

However, if you realize that you are judging, simply notice it. It's not good or bad: it is what is happening. It is easy for us to find ourselves judging. With this practice, you can begin to break out of that pattern. As soon as you notice that you are judging, your judgment will stop. When you are aware of it, you can no longer be caught up in it. This is how the practice of meditation and the presence we experience through it helps us self-correct our subconscious patterns.

An Example of Accepting the Moment and Surrendering

The point of surrender is a key place of transformation for those who suffer. It sure was for me.

My experience of chronic pain—anything that I did not accept in the moment—was that I pushed up against it. I didn't want the moment to be the way it was. I didn't like it. My subconscious reaction was to resist. However, not only was I resisting, but the very act of resisting brought more to resist.

Imagine that you are walking along and a wall is before you. You do not like the wall or accept that it is here. The wall is in your way and you want it to change, but you can't make it go away. You want to get past the wall, but you can't go around it. There is only you and the wall. You want to move forward, but the wall does not move. The solution is to surrender to the wall. As soon as you stop resisting, the wall disappears, and you can once again move forward.

This is a perfect metaphor for what happens when we feel sensation in the body, label it as "bad," try to change it, and finally surrender to the sensation we feel. We accept it as it is. We accept what we are experiencing in the moment.

Here is an experience that brought this lesson home to me. I was feeling overwhelmed. The feeling seemed to rise in front of me like a great black wall. I was afraid of this feeling and the wall it represented, so I chose to resist the sensations I was feeling. The more I resisted, the bigger the wall grew. I felt even more overwhelmed. Finally, I realized that the only thing I could do was stop resisting what I was feeling. It felt like a desperate and brave move on my part, but I just let go of trying to control the situation. As soon as I dropped my fight, the sense of being overwhelmed dissolved. By accepting the moment with all its intense sensation, I found a place of tranquility in surrendering to it.

Suffering is transformed into a place of contentment when we learn to accept what is here in the moment. When we feel intense sensation, we can practice noticing that what we are feeling is a lot of energy. We can remove the spin the mind wants to add by calling all that energy "bad" and trying to change it somehow. We shift suffering into a neutral experience. The sensations we feel may be intense, yet when witnessed without judgment, they feel like a lot of flowing energy.

Imagine that you are trying to fit the whole of the river at the bottom of the Grand Canyon into a hose. Then, in your mind, remove the hose and watch the water flow freely. This is what we do when we try to control the sensations we feel. When we stop trying to control it, we notice that energy changes and becomes free flowing. The body's intelligence will direct that energy into healing energy.

The Power of the Breath in Managing Stress and Chronic Pain

One of the first places to begin effectively managing your stress level is with the power inherent in your breath. The most important thing you do all day to take care of yourself is to breathe fully and consciously.

Your conscious use of the breath is important to your health and healing from the changes that long-term stress and chronic pain cause in the brain. Most of us breathe most of the time in a shallow—even rushed—way. This sends a signal of poor nourishment to the body's cells. Our most core need, for oxygen, is not being met.

Let's look more closely at how this plays out in the body. Normally we breathe in an unconscious, irregular, shallow, and rapid manner. This results in chronic tension and a general unsteadiness. We don't feel rooted and sure in the world, and no wonder—because we are *not* rooted. The lungs supply oxygen and remove carbon dioxide waste from the body, but the lungs also help regulate pH balance, help us excrete water through the exhale, and cool us through the inhale. When we do not breathe fully, using our total lung capacity, our body cannot function properly.

Take this in for a moment: if you laid out the surface area of a pair of adult human lungs, it would cover an area the size of a tennis court. Our lungs need that large surface area to supply our bodies with oxygen, yet most of us live at only about 10 percent of that capacity.

Further, more than half the tiny air sacs that take in air are in the base of the lungs. When we breathe shallowly, we allow carbon dioxide to accumulate there and deny our cells the nourishment they need by not inhaling all the oxygen they need. Those small air sacs, the alveoli, cannot do their job of cleaning out the mucous linings and flushing out toxic waste and irritants that lead to disease and infection.

The power of conscious breathing is that we change that shallow breathing dynamic and turn on the healing power and vitality that the breath holds for us. It calms the effects of a reactive amygdala on our nervous system and so calms us. It helps balance the brain and the nervous system and nourishes the entire body, bringing wellness to every cell.

Using Meditation for Stress Relief

Using meditation, you can find stress relief and turn a life of hustle and bustle into a life of flow. We are so easily caught up in the busyness of life that we tend to push the moment, trying to make it into something that hasn't quite happened. When we are always rushing around, we lose our ability to experience life in the flow.

Meditation is a generic word that means "to quietly and deeply focus inward" as practiced in many traditions. The word springs from the word *dhyana*, which means "one-pointedness of the mind." This is achieved by focusing the mind's attention on one object or image. Meditation is a process of being calm and present in the moment, rather than struggling to change what is happening.

Our reactions to the constant pressures of life can cause chronic stress and chronic pain. Studies have shown that using mindfulness reduces chronic pain. The state of being that is experienced through the practice of mindfulness calms the mind and allows the brain to heal.

People complain that they find meditation boring, and so they dismiss its usefulness to them. This is illuminating to me. It tells me that they are coming right up to the edge of the field of freedom from feeling harried by life.

We are addicted to our excitement, our stimulation, whether it's the rush of adrenaline, the constant activity of our busyness, or the heaviness of depression. We are used to filling our experience with something. We have lost touch with spending any time simply being. Yet, when we are still, we want to fill that stillness, because we are so used to loading the moment with something.

Boredom is a judgment on stillness. Boring is the way in. Boredom is the doorway to our balance and to quieting the mind. It is a gift where we find the power of surrender if we can sit with it long enough. When we can sit with our boredom, allow it to be what it is, and observe it and how we are reacting to it, we discover the neutral mind. What is the value of the neutral mind? We sit without judging our experience, but merely observe it.

How you deal with boredom in meditation is the key to your transformation. Can you stay with the boredom and watch it? Or will you slip back into the old patterns of always wanting to keep a busy and engaged mind and stop attending to your boredom altogether? If you can sit and watch your reaction to the boredom, you will discover that your boredom falls away and you enter a whole other realm, one you cannot access in the busy-minded, thinking world.

The sameness experienced in meditation is the calm dwelling place that you have been trying to reach all along through the hustle and bustle of life. You might think you can rest at the end of all that frantic activity. But wouldn't you rather learn a way of moving through life flowing with the moment instead of fighting with it? The repeated mantra and the cycle of the breath or heartbeat are points of delicious monotony—the opposite of what our busy mind is used to, but just what will bring balance to our lives.

Get curious about expanding beyond your limitations. Ask yourself, *Who will I be without the busyness in my life?* Perhaps you have been pushing for so long, you do not know who you would be without it. It's okay *not* to know. Get curious about not knowing.

Meditation teaches you how to slow down, how to release the concept of time altogether and not fill the moment with anything at all. It reveals that the moment is the reward. You meet it without expectation. When you are fretting about your busy world, time becomes an opponent you engage as if in a battle. You discover that in the meditative space, your concept of time dissolves altogether and you are suspended in an eternal moment.

In meditation, we experience the "nothing," which the mind, our ego, cannot quite wrap itself around. Meditation teaches us how to wait. We discover the secrets hidden in the in-between places, the spaces between thoughts, breaths, and heartbeats. These spaces are where the quietness is beyond imagining. We must discover them through experience.

Nestled in the belly of boredom is the peace you've been seeking for so long.

Meditation holds the reward of being fully consciously aware in the moment. Each moment becomes a discovery, a dynamic learning ground for an ever-unfolding new reality. It teaches us to release our expectations about how things should happen. For the chronically stressed person and chronic pain sufferer, this is a powerful and effective healing tool to ease your life and bring serenity.

The Importance of Self-Care

*Since you alone are responsible for your thoughts,
only you can change them.*

— Paramahansa Yogananda

The concept of self-care is at the core of healing from chronic pain. You must stop running from your pain, from those parts of yourself that are uncomfortable to deal with. As chronic pain has changed the brain, it has also changed the relationship you have with yourself and your spiritual connection. You may have felt victimized by your pain and by your body. You may even have felt that your Higher Power deserted you or punished you. In victimization, we contract and can fall into feeling that self-care is a futile exercise.

Part of healing the changes you undergo when you have experienced chronic pain lies in rising from victimization to empowerment. Take responsibility for your contribution to your pain. Take steps to release old behavior patterns and adopt new ways of being, like staying present and noticing how you feel instead of trying to avoid your pain.

Renew your conscious contact with a power greater and more loving than yourself. Learn to trust in the body's innate ability to heal. Learn to let the healing process take place in its time, instead of trying to make it happen the way and in the time you want it to. Learn to trust your Higher Power and your body, and learn to trust yourself in the process. As you learn to trust yourself to stay present with the things that make you feel uncomfortable, you will begin to relax deeply, perhaps for the first time since you can remember.

Your commitment to your healing includes bringing your self-care to a new level. You will be transformed by the shift from feeling victimized by your circumstances to being empowered through conscious, purposeful living. You may have intense physical sensations, yet you can learn to carefully and consciously craft the meaning you make of those sensations. In the end, it isn't the sensations that cause suffering and distress but the story and meaning you make of them. Drop the label you use for your condition and simply feel it. Any meaning you give it, if you give one at all, is neutral. For example, "I'm feeling tension and pressure in my head" instead of "I'm having another migraine headache."

When you stay in the present moment and in neutral, you use two of the most important self-care tools you have. When you use them, you are centered in the heart of the Healing Field.

Let your self-care become a daily and even moment-to-moment practice of conscious choosing, patience, compassion, forgiveness, and full acceptance of yourself. Become fiercely devoted and radically committed to your self-care as you find your way toward cracking the code of chronic pain and discovering a thriving life.

About Blocks and Limitations

To use a baseball analogy, life throws us all kinds of balls. We hit some out of the park, hit some fouls, and miss others altogether. We can get discouraged. Remember the negative thinking habit I spoke of earlier? It will put up all kinds of blocks for us on our healing journey. One way to look at a block is as something that gets in our way that we must figure out how to push through. That approach might work, but it comes at a cost.

We push through the world like we are pushing back a river. We are the ones who suffer with this approach. Everything becomes an almost insurmountable battle.

Consider your perspective on the whole situation. In our negative thinking, a block is a "no," and we shut down in response to it. We can give up trying altogether. The second Aquarian Sutra says, "There's a way through every block." Consider this: the block is there to test your mettle. The block is there to spur your creativity. The block is there to help you magnify your courage. The block is there as a marker on your path.

So, the next time you face a block in your life, bow to it and say thank you, for it is a powerful teacher. As much as you want to get around, through, or beyond the block, it is in your approach to and way of dealing with the block where the magic truly lies.

You can move through blocks with the sheer will of your ego, but this is a circuitous route, and will no doubt bring pain and suffering. Or you can move through it with the aid of your Higher Power, listening to your inner knowing to guide you. This approach moves us in the direction of the flow-through instead of trying to "push the river."

In recovering from chronic pain, find the flow. Find the path that is the smoother one. We have been so used to "pushing through" life just to survive that we have become our own enemy. We are so accustomed to resistance that we tend to meet the world carrying the frequency of resistance, of "pushing through," of seeing everything as a fight just to move forward.

I am advocating for cultivating gentleness as you meet the world. When you feel yourself tightening up as you go through your day, pause for a moment. Breathe. Ask your Higher Power for help and guidance. Listen. You will be guided through. How can I say such a thing? Because I have lived this. I have found that when I meet the world with more tenderness and more listening, and less pushing, it becomes an easier place to navigate.

There is a sweet-spot flow zone hiding in every block you meet. Take the time to find it. Your life will become sweeter in the process, and you will heal.

Your Attention in Healing Unhealthy Habits

We have all kinds of habits. Most of the time they run as unconscious programs in the background of our lives. We can take an action that brings us comfort, but if we are not paying attention, it can lead to self-destructive behavior. For example, when you're stressed, do you unconsciously seek food for comfort? I am especially drawn to carbohydrates, sugar, and fats: chocolate is my guilty pleasure. But the next thing I know, my food choices have gone awry, and I am stressed in a whole new way. What began as self-soothing turns into self-destruction.

I have been using unhealthy food choices as a calming tool ever since I can remember. It is an example of what happens when we are no longer consciously making choices. There are many other strategies I can use to manage stress, and I have a support system when I need it.

For me, it's all about fear and safety. When I'm uncomfortable and my fear alarm goes off, I no longer feel safe. To calm the fear, I automatically turn to the closest thing I associate with a sense of safety. The urge to eat something that has a dopamine reward associated with it, like a sugary food, is almost inevitable. I know this about myself, so I keep such foods out of my reach. That way if I want something like a cupcake or some ice cream, I must go out and search for it. Between my craving for sugar and the safety it represents, I become conscious of my actions. Once I am aware of what is driving me from within, I make a healthier conscious choice to deal with my stress.

It's all a trick of the mind! None of it is real. It's just a part of me that wants to stay safe and comfortable.

We all have our little habits: smoking, alcohol, drugs, sex, food, gambling, playing the victim, negative thinking. Whatever your pattern is, shifting it to a new way of being in the world can bring up a lot of resistance, fear, and self-doubt. Know that your awareness and the focus of your attention are the tools to transforming that pattern into a healthier one.

Nutrition and Hydration

This is not to sound preachy. I am as susceptible to enticing "junk" food as the next person. With that said, I offer this: food is information for the body. What we feed it has a direct effect on how we will feel after we eat it and on the body's ability to heal itself. Junk food is junk information, and so does not help healing. Healthy food has healing properties and is of paramount importance if we are to heal. Our food choices come down to this simple question: is this food choice going to help me heal or is it going to add to the junk load of information I am trying to clear in the first place? The answer reflects our commitment to ourselves about healing.

In my case, some of my chronic pain was caused by my body's sensitivity to inflammatory foods. We now have the advantage of being able to test for food sensitivities and allergies. I investigated mine and used the results to tailor my diet so that it is as close to optimal as possible. I further fine-tuned my diet by learning about my base metabolic type with the help of Dr. Philip Goglia.

I cannot overstate the importance of proper hydration. As a chronic pain patient, I was underweight and dehydrated by medication. I was always thirsty. My lips cracked frequently. My digestive tract was paralyzed by both the medication and poor hydration. This condition only added to my pain and stress levels.

I learned something in treatment that surprised me. I had access to three meals each day, yet I was often hungry between meals. I drank water to quell my hunger pangs and noticed that the food cravings disappeared. I discovered that I had been confusing hunger with thirst. It seemed like a subtle difference, yet it was profound.

I learned that when I drank more water, I felt better—noticeably better. I started drinking water frequently during the day and learned to take a water bottle with me everywhere I went.

Sleep Hygiene

The chronic pain "lifestyle" holds so much stress that sleep is often elusive or sometimes even absent. Our nervous system is rattled to the core, and our brain has undergone concurrent changes. I cannot say enough about how important high-quality sleep is to the healing process. Do whatever you can to ensure the best sleep you can. Letting anything or anyone get in the way of a peaceful night's sleep, and as much as you can get, sabotages your healing. Take sleep seriously.

When You Still Can't Sleep

What do you do when you wake up in the middle of the night and can't get back to sleep? All you want to do is sleep, yet it eludes you. Everything seems to close in on you: yesterday's chores left undone, worrying about tomorrow, fretting about functioning without enough sleep.

You would rather be anywhere else but in this moment. I understand. I have lived this moment. It is a time of rebellion against our being. Against the night itself. It is a time of aloneness. It is a time of pain. You are pushing against the moment. You try again, pushing harder this time. No matter how hard you try, pushing doesn't work. You just want rest, if only for a moment.

This is a turning point. Will you be able to find a point of surrender and accept the moment? Or will you continue to fight with your assessment that the moment is painful?

If you stay in the battle, it will overpower you, because you are looking outside yourself, thinking that because the reason for it is "out there," you should seek a solution "out there." That is relapse territory. You must heed yourself. Where is your attention? Look to Step 1 and your spiritual program. Realize you are powerless in this moment. Recognize that surrender is an option. Realize you don't ever have to use drugs again. Turn your fear, your fight, your pain over to the Higher Power of your understanding. Release your worries and anything else that is uncomfortable. You are no longer alone, because you see that your Higher Power is with you. Learn to lie still with the sleeplessness. Discover the quietude and become still in this place. This is the result of all the hours you spent in meetings, on a yoga mat, reading the literature, working with your sponsor and the steps. It's paying great dividends. It's saving your life. Even if sleep proves elusive for this one night, you will learn the real power in this moment. You have surrendered to all of it. You are free from using. You are free from aloneness. You are free from the pain. In realizing your powerlessness, you reconnect with your Higher Power and drift in the everlasting moment, unfettered. Free.

How to Unlock Your Healing Potential

Practice these tips as often as you can:

- Become the witness to and observer of your experience.
- Decide where you are going to put your attention.
- Radically change your diet to one as healthy as possible.
- Take control of your health.
- Follow your intuition.
- Use herbs and supplements as suggested by a doctor.

- Release suppressed emotions.
- Increase positive emotions.
- Embrace social support.
- Deepen your spiritual connection.
- Have a strong reason for living.
- Believe the diagnosis, but not the prognosis.

A Final Word on Self-Care

This business of self-care: I cannot stress it enough. You did the best you could to take care of yourself, but often felt it wasn't enough, because you were still in chronic pain. You can get in the habit of believing that self-care is not worth the effort to change your old ways and develop new, healthier ways of living.

You must believe in yourself, and you must guard this belief against all doubt.

You must believe in your body's miraculous ability to heal, and you must guard this belief against all doubt.

Develop a fierce commitment to yourself.

Curry ways to gentle how you meet and move in the world.

Pushing through the world is no longer an option as you move into recovery from chronic pain and active addiction.

You now have tools to help calm yourself and find peace in whatever storms life brings. It is up to you to pick up the tools and use them.

Make your practice of self-care impeccable. Be meticulous in designing the rituals in your life that ensure the highest quality of care you can give yourself.

Speak to yourself as if you were speaking to your best friend and to your child, because you are speaking to both.

Come to terms with your doubts and fears. Realize that they are there for a reason. Do what you can to tame your negative thinking habit.

As a chronic pain sufferer, you may doubt that you are worthy of living a life free from pain, where you do not have to constantly push through the world, where your best effort is more than enough. Your worthiness was never an issue; the stories you built up around it are. Take note of what you are saying to yourself about your worthiness. If you doubt your worthiness, rescript your story around it. This is deep work. It may take some time. Every moment of this work is sacred. Please stick with it, for if worthiness is an issue for you, here is where you can heal a critical part of what started you on the path to chronic pain in the first place.

Give yourself—all parts of yourself—unconditional love. No matter what.

Finding a New Way to Live: The Elements of a Daily Practice

*The magic spark of healing lives in our showing up
and stepping up to the work.*

— Elizabeth Kipp

Quieting the mind is the single most important requirement of a daily practice. Anything that promotes moving toward the stillness within us fits this need. You might ask, "What about feeding the soul?" I say we must begin with quieting the mind so that we may tune in to the limitless field of awareness that is the soul. It is only from this space of consciousness that we can hear the soul speak to us. When we find that silent pool deep in ourselves, we discover what a rich Healing Field resides there. We find answers, lots of answers, maybe even most of them. We find a sublime peace, and isn't peace what we've been going for all along?

Other critical prerequisites to a daily practice are showing up to it and being willing to accept all that the practice brings to you. No matter what your mind might offer as a reason to turn away from it, the act of stepping into practice releases part of the power of a practice. That is, all you have to do once you get to the practice is do the practice. You can do it with heart. You can do it with anger. You can do it like an automaton from sheer memory. Any way you slice it, so long as you do the work of the practice, you will succeed and benefit.

Remember that you are changing things on a molecular and biochemical level as you do your practice. Continuing to practice is critical. When we learn something new, we create new neural pathways in the brain. However, without repetition, these new pathways degrade quickly. To build a lasting new neural network in the brain, we must repeat the behavior. Remember how hard it seems when you are learning something new? This is because you are literally creating. It takes energy, and then reviewing the new material again and again, to set it in your memory. Once you have memorized it, it is easier to access that information. This is because you have established the new neural pathway for it in the brain. The creating takes work. Have patience with your practice as your body does this miraculous work for you.

The breath is the bridge through it all. As you do your practice, allow what comes up for you to arise and flow through you without judgment. Regardless of how you are getting through your practice, you will emerge victorious, because you are present and steady in the breath.

You have lived with chronic pain long enough for changes to occur in your brain. To heal, you must bring new ways of living into play that help reverse these changes. Further, since you have experienced so much isolation in your suffering, it is imperative that you incorporate a spiritual element into your life or put greater emphasis on it. This will deepen your ability to forgive and restore your sense of being connected to the body, others, and your Higher Power, whatever that is for you.

Practices that are simple, profound, and deeply healing include qigong, meditation, and yoga; releasing shame, guilt, and judgment by deepening your compassion and cultivating forgiveness; nurturing a sense of gratitude; and renewing your awareness of your connection to nature and a power greater and more loving than yourself. These practices speak directly to the union of mind, body, and spirit, something chronic pain sufferers have lost. Each practice is a vehicle to quieting the mind and accessing that peaceful, soulful space within you.

Hear me! These practices work! They have helped me move, dissolve, and clear a lifetime of pain. They bring relief to anxiety, grief, the weight of sadness, and other kinds of suffering—and they do so without pharmaceuticals. We are blessed to have been granted access to these tools.

When we turned to medication or other substances or activities in the past to ease our pain, our search was in earnest. We were lost. Those avenues may have offered a short-term solution, but they were not a long-term one. And it is an illusion that they helped at all. So long as we are covering our pain, so long as we turn away from ourselves, we are only adding to our pain load.

Chronic pain changes our relationship to ourselves all the way to our soul. Our trust in our body and in ourselves is shaken to the core. Solutions that speak to these changes are the ones we are looking for. Those are the ones that will raise you from the ashes of your life and grow your wings so that you can rise like the proverbial phoenix.

Why We Practice

After I got clean from all the pain and anti-anxiety medication I had been on for so long and my physical pain cleared, I came alive with sensation. I was also almost overwhelmed by the pattern of negative thinking that was running rampant through my mind.

However, I knew I had a tendency toward negativity and that it was part of the patterning in the old neural network in my brain. I knew about the brain's plasticity, its ability to rewire itself in response to changing behavioral conditions. I was at the beginning of my recovery and in the process of literally building a new neural network. This takes time. I would have to eat healthy food, drink plenty of water, and stimulate my body in such a way that I would grow new neurons and dendritic pathways in my brain to nurture and "program" new behaviors.

I had to take actions that would help nurture my body's natural healing ability, since a big part of the healing lay in developing a new neural network in the brain. Again, the repetitive actions of a daily practice provide this.

Your practice is your vehicle for transformation. In my view, the real magic of a practice is that all that is required is to show up and do the practice. The body takes its cue from you and does all the building and healing for you. That is how strong our willingness can be in determining the success of our recovery. The magic spark of healing lives in your showing up and stepping up to the work.

Where is your devotion? Does it live in your commitment to your healing?

With the ego being the beast that it is, your commitment to healing must be so strong that you desire it more than anything, beyond the yapping, arguing, and protesting that the ego will insist on doing.

Do your practice even, and especially, when you don't want to do it. Do your practice even when you have forgotten why you are doing it.

Each time you come into your practice, you come back to yourself. You recommit to your practice, and more importantly, you recommit to yourself.

Ultimately this is why we practice: we say yes again and again to finding a new way to live. Our practice builds this habit of saying yes to our healing and ourselves.

Elements of a Practice

These are the elements of a practice.

Show up and be willing.

Quiet the mind. We are using techniques to quiet the mind. Healing arises from the place of presence and a quieted mind. It's that simple. It doesn't have to take a lot of time.

Develop a witness consciousness. By staying in the role of witness, you will transcend your tendency to live in that self-critical, negative pattern of thinking. By being a witness to your thoughts, you will develop the clarity to see yourself when you get dragged back into your old habits by your ego. Simply notice this phenomenon. The act of noticing it, of being aware of it, will bring you out of it.

Do not bring any shame or judgment to your practice. There is no need to defend or criticize yourself. You are simply in touch with an old part of yourself. It served you in the past, but it is not needed now. Acknowledge its presence and stay present, noticing what is arising. That negativity will self-correct as you remain present.

Drop expectation. This is an exercise in presence, in noticing. Again, you are the witness. Just notice what is arising within you. Notice the energy within.

Nurture your awareness. Choose awareness instead of negative thinking or wanting things to be the way you want them to be. Meet the practice and yourself where you are—right here, right now.

You may not understand everything, and that's okay. There is a lot more intelligence within us than we realize. Our practice helps bring this out. We have the experience of a vaster space inside of us, and vast intelligence to go with it. This experience is not something the mind can identify, categorize, or otherwise easily reference. That's okay. Let go of the need for the mind to understand. If you must give it a name, call it "energy." Keep it simple.

The most important relationship we have is with our self. We come face-to-face with ourselves regularly in our practice, quite the opposite of what we did when we were suffering in active addiction.

Sadhana

The idea of *sadhana* (homework) is to develop a daily practice that sustains you. It is usually done first thing in the morning and helps you begin your day in a purposeful, grounded way. You support it by showing up. It supports you by grounding your awareness of your connection to your Higher Power and by helping you develop an internal discipline. It includes bowing to a power greater and more loving than yourself, conscious breathing, and attuning your body to a healthy vibrational frequency through some form of prayer, which can include a mantra. It nurtures your healing and your transformation. It helps give you a sense of feeling grounded throughout the day. It allows your joy to blossom.

It can be challenging to get up a little earlier just so you can do your practice. I understand. Everyone I know who has a daily practice understands. Here's the thing: the rewards of rising to the challenge of doing this practice are well worth your effort and more.

I work a physical practice of yoga and/or qigong, an emotional and spiritual practice that reminds me that I am not in charge of the universe. My Higher Power runs the show. I remind myself every morning when I bow to the Creator what the power structure is and where I fit in it.

I begin every morning anew. This planet has always lived by a twenty-four-hour cycle. All living organisms evolved in this same cycle. It is our reality. We recognize and honor this relationship when we begin again each day. Our daily practice is the perfect recipe for reviewing and renewing our relationship with Creator, Earth, and ourselves.

The discipline you develop will sustain you so that whatever happens, you can always rise to meet it. It will allow you to have the long-lived experience of moving out of *doing* all the time and into more *being*, becoming aware of the energy field, the life force pulsing within you.

Gratitude and the Gratitude Journal

Practicing gratitude is foundational for healing and for living a thriving life. It is easy to become swept up in the role of victim when you experience chronic pain. You are stressed, and you become anxious. It is easy to compare the present moment with the past and then project into the future: "I feel this pain, just like I felt it before, and it will be just like this in the future." You can lock yourself into a painful cycle of stress and anxiety just by believing that sentence. You can become lost in your victimhood, almost hold yourself hostage in the belief that you will always feel like this, because you have felt this way for so long. Part of healing and living beyond the stress and anxiety you experience with the cycle of chronic pain is in shifting out of the frequency of lack and victimhood and into the frequency of abundance and recovery through the practice of gratitude.

Studies have shown the effect gratitude has on relieving pain and rewiring the brain to help heal the changes chronic pain brings. Practicing gratitude helps regulate levels of dopamine, a neurotransmitter that helps regulate movement, attention, learning, and emotional responses. It helps fill us with an expansive vitality and so reduces our experience of pain.

Gratitude is part of what vibrates within the frequency of abundance. If you are focusing on how stressed you are, you get hung up in the feeling of being stressed. But if you focus instead on how blessed you are, you shift your focus to a whole other energy state and open to the frequency of gratitude, the baseline in the frequency of abundance.

Using the power of gratitude, you can stay present in the Healing Field. You have dropped your pattern of slipping back into the past and projecting what your future will be. You have stopped your voice of worry, since that voice lives in the future and you are staying present. The anxiety associated with worry dissolves. Your stress is often wrapped up in your fretting about how things could be, yet you are not even there yet.

When you remove yourself from projecting into the future, and even forecasting what your future will be, you have a different experience of living, one that is calmer and more peaceful. You are living in the moment, not in the past or the future.

I begin the day powerfully when I wake up by saying thank you to my Higher Power. I have a gratitude journal where I write down three things I am grateful for each day. I hope you will try this practice for at least forty days and see what happens. It takes thirty days to break a habit and begin building a new one. The forty-day practice helps better seal the new pattern into our lives. I have done a number of forty-day practices and found them very helpful in shifting from an old, unhealthy behavior to a new, healthier one. When we focus on the blessings in life, and realize that all life is a blessing, we shift into the frequency of gratitude, which lives in the Healing Field.

Qigong

Qigong has roots that go back five thousand years in the East. I was introduced to it in Dr. Przekop's Pain Management Program. Even in my weakened state, I was able to do these movements. In this practice we use the breath, energy, and presence to help quiet the mind and enable us to get to a place where we can heal body, mind, and spirit. We use the breath and energy to clear energetic blocks. We learn to view the inside of the body as energy and allow ourselves to become present and quiet, thereby allowing the body optimal conditions in which to heal. This practice takes us right into the Healing Field.

Yoga

The first line in the first chapter of the *Yoga Sutras of Patanjali* is "Atha-Yoganusasanum," which translates as "Now the discipline of Yoga is explained." The first word of the sutra, *atha*, means "now." Another way of interpreting this verse is that yoga is now. Practicing yoga brings us into the present moment.

Why yoga as a path through chronic pain and its ensuing addiction, the endless shadow of negativity, and the suffering?

Out in the world we look to food, media, sex, drugs, money, power, and prestige—anything to control, avoid, and distract ourselves from the uncomfortable. Our spirit longs for something. We feel a constant restlessness in our body. Our mind races. We cannot escape, no matter how we might try. We lose ourselves in treasured memories or dreams about our future and miss what's happening now. We look anywhere but here, the present moment.

We finally realize we are on a fool's errand. Whatever we are searching or longing for eludes us. There comes a time when we clearly see how utterly lost we are. We stop and stand on the brink. We have nowhere left to go but here. And now yoga. Yoga means "to yoke mind, body, and spirit." Yoga is a way through chronic pain. It gets us to stay here in the now. It requires our attention in the present. In chronic pain there is chaos, angst, and suffering. In yoga we find peace, quiet, and contentment.

Mantra

A mantra is a mentally or vocally repeated word or phrase used as a form of meditation. The use of mantra helps bring us into the present moment. Being present is reason enough to use mantra in a practice. The word *mantra* means "mind wave" or "projection." In Sanskrit it means "mental liberation: to bring light to the mind."

Our mind is constantly barraged by thousands of thoughts. Mantra helps us calm the mind and focus it by using the sound of our voice, combined with our breath, and reciting the root sounds of ancient language linked into the Earth. Mantra is spoken aloud in some traditions, but not all. For instance, Transcendental

Meditation uses mantras, but they are said silently rather than out loud.

Sound is a form of energy that exists in a wave that travels at a certain frequency. It has structure and inherent power. Mantra is sound that affects patterns of the mind and the brain. It has both physical and metaphysical effects on the human psyche. We use mantra as a sound meditation to shift our consciousness.

For example, mantra can be used to help navigate feelings of grief or sadness. As chronic pain sufferers or people in recovery from chronic pain, we feel our emotions but find ourselves swimming in a sea of feelings. We have learned to not judge emotions as "good" or "bad," yet they have their own energetic frequency. Using mantra appropriately can help us navigate those emotions with more ease. It allows us to moderate the energy frequency we are experiencing. It helps us "surf" that sea of emotions more easily.

The effects of meditation on the brain have been heavily researched. One study showed that 92 percent of respondents who used meditation, including mantra, said it helped them manage their stress more effectively; 91 percent found that meditation helped them build emotional stability.

My own personal experience with mantra is that it helps me stay steady when I might otherwise feel unsure of myself during a great swell of emotion. So, the practice of mantra in meditation helps us build our capacity for resilience.

Get Outside

Not surprisingly, studies show that when we spend time in nature, we are better able to relax and rest. The brain heals when it experiences nature. For those of us recovering from chronic pain, our time in nature helps bring us into the present moment, thereby curtailing our tendencies to ruminate and catastrophize. Specifically, research reveals that the subgenual prefrontal cortex, a part of the brain associated with negative thinking, has less blood flow after we spend time outdoors. This part of the brain is quieter, which allows us to experience increased feelings of well-being.

There is something deeply primal and fulfilling about being outside in the elements. We get a direct experience of the Higher Power of our understanding. We are tuned in. We leave our modern high-tech way of being behind and get "in the zone" where we humans lived not that many years ago. We bring in our sense of being connected to the All That Is. We move from the state of "doing" to the state of "being."

Your time outside is indeed a living mindful meditation. Tap into the awesomeness of these natural external cues that then allow you to more easily access your inner awesomeness. (I know that doesn't sound very scientific, but nonetheless, that's what happens.) The power of healing that being in nature brings into your recovery cannot be underestimated. I encourage you to add this potent mantra to your list—"get outside"—and apply it liberally each day.

Community Support

It's important to be in a community of like-minded people who are healing from chronic pain. When we band together and share our experience, strength, and hope in coping with and healing from chronic pain, we vastly increase the odds that we will succeed in finding a way of life free from suffering. Chronic pain sufferers live in isolation; we get disconnected from each other and from ourselves and forget our connection to the Higher Power of our understanding. Community is an essential part of the healing process, for the therapeutic value of one chronic pain patient helping another is beyond measure. It is my fervent hope that you will join in community to find support and, just as important, nurture your sense of purpose by being of service to others.

You can begin with Narcotics Anonymous or Chronic Pain Anonymous. You can find Refuge Recovery, SMART Recovery, or Recovery 2.0. You might be able to find a Yoga 12-Step Recovery (Y12SR) meeting. There are others. Look in your community and find like-minded people with whom you can share your healing journey. Find a mentor who has been through the process of healing from chronic pain. You can find help working the twelve steps by finding a sponsor through one of the twelve-step fellowships.

Remember These Basics

Drop the effort and the expectation. Just show up and do the work. Let the practice meet you where you are. So long as you show up, the practice will work its power, regardless of how you are. Do not expect anything. Do the work of the practice the best you can. Do not judge yourself. Stay in the neutral mind as much as possible. If your mind wanders, just bring it back.

Focus within.

Realize that the love you are looking for is already within you, just the way you are in this moment. It is not a key you lost somewhere. It is right here. It has always been here. It is the very core of life itself. Everything is being held in love, even the pain. Once you embrace the pain, you'll find that there is always love. It has always been there. In the beginning it may be a choice you need to make, to choose love as a visceral experience. The heartbeat, the breath, the awareness. We do not understand all of it. Yet here we are. Here. From two cells to who we are in this moment, the drive is toward growth. This is love. You don't need to go away from yourself; you come closer to yourself. It will wait for you. It is always here. It will always be here. Come back to yourself. There is no effort here. There is only love.

Life will test you. It will expand your limits. It will challenge your beliefs. It doesn't really matter which way you turn, or where you hang your hat or rest your head. You are always there to meet yourself. The moment brings itself, and you decide how you are going to meet it. You can want for more and get lost in and even consumed by that yearning, or you can settle into it. You can wrestle with what you find in the present moment and try to change the immutable, or you can accept what is here and ultimately find peace. It's your decision. That is how powerful your choices are.

A practice doesn't expect you to show up all happy and smiling. It doesn't have any expectations at all. A practice holds you to one promise and one promise only: to show up. You don't have to have it all together. You can be a simpering mess. You do not have to come with your glow on. You can show up all prickly with confusion or infused with sadness. A practice holds space for it all. In return for the presence a practice brings, it asks only that you show up and bring your own presence. It has this miraculous way of blessing whatever you bring into it. As a result, you grow and are transformed.

Meet yourself where you are. Whatever it is that you are feeling in this moment is your truth, no matter what others say. Love yourself where you are. I know it can be hard. Give yourself a break. You are a powerful being. Full of grit. Full of brilliance. You know—the star stuff that you are.

- Get enough rest and sleep.
- Eat well and stay well hydrated.
- Get outside.
- Be grateful.
- Help others.
- Self-love has no conditions. It's right here, right now.
- Continue to do your practice every day . . . for the rest of your life.

The 12 Steps of Wellness

*Do the work every day for the rest of your life—and you
will live a thriving life beyond the reach of suffering.*

— Elizabeth Kipp

Courage and the Chronic Pain Sufferer/Addict

When you have known pain to the point where you dread
it coming back, you have entered the dragon's lair and
felt the heat of its fire. The pain has cowed you, shocked you,
terrified you. You begin to experience life from a place of worry
and anticipation.

*I see that there is a dragon here. I have felt its fire before, and it
is fierce and terrible. When will I feel that fire again? (Mind you, not
what if I feel it again? but when will I feel it again?) When will the
great pain dragon unleash its punishing flame of fire again? And will
I survive it next time?*

These are the very real thoughts of a chronic pain sufferer
or addict. Ask anyone who has dealt with chronic migraine
headaches, for example. Or anyone who has felt the relentless
insistence of wanting relief from the unendurable.

You have been dwelling in dread for a long time. It can be a
place of almost complete hopelessness.

You can see the incredible courage of someone in chronic pain.
Somewhere deep inside of us we must know the healing power
and magic that lives in there. We may not be able to see it. It may
not be conscious, but if we didn't know it was in there on some
level, our courage would have dried up long ago.

Yet that thread between our dread and the inner knowing
that sustains our courage is the bridge that keeps us connected

to ourselves and our Higher Power. We became isolated from the world, from our friends, from ourselves in many ways. Yet through all of it we have this connection, even with the slimmest of threads between the dire and hope. It may be subconscious, yet it remains. It is waiting for us to awaken. It is the sweet healing voice of our Higher Power turned down to a mere whisper in the confusion of our suffering.

We get attached to our dread in a predictable yet twisted way. It becomes so familiar that to drop it, to let it go, would mean giving up our very identity. Imagine how much courage it takes to let go of your identity.

Yet this is the kind of courage that an addict and chronic pain sufferer musters to awaken to their true identity. This is the kind of courage it takes to decide to put down the drugs and try something completely different.

Think about this the next time you meet someone who tells you they are a recovering addict or recovering chronic pain sufferer. They have entered the dragon's lair, felt its fire, dreaded its fury, and found a way to transmute that fire into a waterfall.

The struggle of the chronic pain sufferer and those in recovery is real but optional, depending on how long we want to hang on to our stories and beliefs (and so long as we aren't lost in the mind). The transformation to our healing is epic in nature. We do our practices because we want to feel okay and because we know the dread we would be in if we didn't—and we are incredibly grateful to have such tools.

Healing happens on its own terms once we have put ourselves on its path. Walking the line of the distinctly uncomfortable in our life of recovery and resisting the temptation to numb out or let it rule us—or I should say, overrule us—accepting this as part of who we are: here is a piece of learning how to live our recovery without controlling everything in sight.

There is much information in this book. I have done my best to lay out the landscape of the Mind Field, the battlefield of chronic pain. I have described the Healing Field and how to access it. I have included exercises to guide you into the felt experience of the Healing Field.

In conclusion, here are the golden breadcrumbs that lead us through chronic pain into the Healing Field and into a thriving life. I developed these with Peter Przekop in the last weeks of his life, based on the foundation he set out in his book and my practical application of it.

The 12 Steps of Wellness

Here are the 12 Steps of Wellness.

1. None of us were born to suffer.
2. We all have the ability to heal.
3. Love with all your heart.
4. Get real about your healing.
5. Commit to your healing.
6. Do the work it takes to heal.
7. Do the work every day.
8. Get real about your healing. (In case you missed it the first time, it's that important!)
9. Never let anyone or anything get in the way of your healing.
10. Love yourself fiercely and without reservation.
11. Accept what is.
12. Be grateful for all that comes your way, and more will be revealed.

Do the work every day for the rest of your life and you will live a thriving life beyond the reach of suffering.

Self-Reflection Questions and Exercises

Chapter 3

Self-Reflection Questions

To heal, we must face what we are believing and feeling about our pain.

- What beliefs do you have about your pain?
  - Do you believe that there is something "wrong" with you or that you are "broken"?
  - Do you wonder if you will ever get better?
  - Do you believe you will always be in pain?
- What do you believe about the possibilities for your healing?
- What assumptions are you making about your condition?
- Are these assumptions true, or are they just that— assumptions?
- Are you willing to change your current approach to your healing?
- Who would you be without your pain? Describe how you would feel in the absence of pain.
- What would become possible for you without your pain?

Chapter 4

Self-Reflection Questions

Ask yourself these questions:

- What is the story I am telling myself about what I am feeling?
- Is that story true?
- Is it my truth or a truth that I have created?

- Is it an empowering story, or does it lock me into the cycle of chronic pain?

Remember, anger and resistance lock in your pain. Think of your resistance to what you are feeling. Imagine you are in a straitjacket and that the more you struggle, the tighter it gets. That is what resistance does to us.

- How committed am I to my health?
- Am I fighting for my beliefs about my situation more than I am fighting for my health, or is it the other way around?
- How can I rewrite the story I am telling myself to help me rise out of old behavior patterns into a new way of living beyond chronic pain?

Chapter 5

Exercise: Forgive Yourself

You can learn to accept what you are feeling by forgiving yourself for all the judgment you have been holding against yourself. You are human. Release yourself from the bondage and limitation of judgment. If you are having feelings you don't like and are ashamed of yourself for feeling them, forgive yourself.

Love is about being able to hold all of it, the dark and the light, within you. The judgment and interpretation around the parts that you don't want to experience spin you right into the cycle of suffering and chronic pain.

Can you make peace with what is beneath that which is making you angry, shameful, and wanting to deny what you are experiencing—and move forward?

Make peace, forgive, and embrace all of who you are, and deepen your self-love.

You are your life partner.

Make peace with yourself and discover a thriving life beyond the grip of chronic pain.

Exercise: Acceptance and Equanimity

Here is a mindfulness exercise you can use to train yourself to observe in an accepting and more neutral, nonjudgmental way. This meditation is particularly helpful to someone healing their brain from chronic pain. It teaches us to accept every stimulus that comes into our sensory field equally. In other words, we hear, see, smell, sense, touch, and taste all that is in our awareness and accept all these stimuli equally. It is simple to explain and experience, but it is not necessarily easy.

Let me give you an example from my own equanimity meditation practice.

I am lying down on my bed. I can feel the back of my body on the sheets and the covers touching the top of my body. I notice those sensations as I feel them. My eyes are closed, so I see darkness. I notice the darkness. I smell food cooking in the kitchen; I notice the aroma. My tongue tastes the neutral taste of water; I notice the taste. I hear a high-pitched ringing in my ears; then I hear someone walking. I notice these sounds. I do not make any attempt to change my experience by trying to block out or "push against" my experience.

The practice gets a little trickier as I hear a vacuum cleaner being turned on. In my peaceful state, my first reaction is to tense up at this increase in sensory input. If I were to judge this experience now, I might silently say to myself, *I do not like this sound.* In this practice, the idea is to accept *all* input without judging any of it one way or the other, as neither pleasant nor unpleasant.

This is valuable because it trains us away from judging our experience. When we were in chronic pain, we judged the intense sensations we were feeling as "bad" and tried to alter our experience to get away from or dull the sensations we were feeling. Our attempt to change our sensory input is an active state. In this meditation practice, we practice remaining passive and learn to "be" with whatever we are experiencing. Practicing this helps retrain the nervous system to be less reactive to stimuli and reset our previously overworked stress response to a normal level. Calming our nervous system in this way also helps us rest our adrenal glands, which in a chronic pain sufferer are most often in a state of exhaustion.

Self-Reflection Questions

Here are a few action steps to help guide your experience of trading the power of control for the healing power of acceptance:

- You are holding your pain and cannot get rid of it (you've already tried to do it but haven't been successful). Consider releasing your belief that you must hold it.
- Practice mindfulness by releasing your need to control your situation. Do not judge or analyze your experience. Just allow yourself to *be* in your experience.
- Do not compare your healing or your perception of it to anyone else's experience.
- Allow yourself to be exactly who you are, as you are, in the moment, without judgment.
- Practice this every day.

Exercise: Rescript Your Inner Critic
and Cultivate Self-Compassion

We make mistakes. We may feel like we bumble through life. We fall and we get back up again. On the way to getting back up, we can do a good job of beating ourselves up for falling in the first place. Whatever physical injury may have resulted from the fall is often nothing compared with the emotional battering we give ourselves. The drive for perfection and the misconception that we *can* be perfect do not tend to serve us in a healthy way. Indeed, if that drive is strong enough, it can lead us straight into stress, anxiety, and a cycle of chronic pain.

We live in a culture of paradox in many ways. For instance, I was raised in a family where "right" and "wrong" were clearly defined. At school there were right or wrong answers, and we were graded accordingly. In the world of computers, there is "on" and "off"—another right or wrong area in our lives. When we press the wrong keystroke on a computer, the computer software doesn't work the way we intended because we have inadvertently asked it to turn "off." Gray areas where mistakes are encouraged and nourished as doors of discovery instead of eliciting a response of "You got it wrong (again)" just don't fit in the academic world. It is a paradox for us to then shift from that perfectionist kind of thinking and discipline to a way of living that opens us up to trial and error as a fact of life. It is no wonder we are confused and feel frustration and anxiety.

When we bring our awareness to this situation and realize that our inner critic is working overtime in an area where it doesn't even belong, we can make a shift.

Exercise: Taming Your Inner Critic

When our inner critic gets to be this influential in our life, it's time for a makeover. I will take you through the process I used to tame my inner critic.

- *I made a decision to change.* I realized one day that I was so tired of the heavy weight I felt every time I heard the voice of my inner critic that *I wanted to make a change*—once and for all.
- *I asked myself a question. What can I do to effect lasting change and shift how my inner critic shows up for me?* I realized that this inner-critic voice was in some ways a helpful one and that it would always be with me in some way. Knowing and accepting this, I decided to reassign the role of my inner critic, specifically in the way she spoke to me.
- *The makeover.* First, I had to really get a handle on exactly who I was working with. I sat quietly and sensed all that I could about her. What did she look like? What did she wear,

and how did she hold herself in the world? What did she sound like? What kind of mood was she in? What was she feeling? The answers were quite revealing to me. Through answering these questions, I was able to really understand this inner persona much better than I ever had before.

I imagined my inner critic as standing about seven feet tall (to my actual five feet four inches). She wore the black robes of a Supreme Court justice and held a steady, sullen, and stern gaze everywhere she looked as she lorded it over the world, judging all within her reach. Her hair was pulled up into a tight bun. Her face was ashen from not ever being out in the sun. She smelled musty, and like mothballs. She never smiled and always had a negative and critical comment about everything, whether asked for or not. She always came off as serious—and she was relentless.

Well, looking at that powerful personality, it's no wonder I felt heavy and uncomfortable every time I heard her voice! Now my job was to reassign her to a new position altogether. Again, I asked myself, *How would you like her to be?* It was my choice, after all. I was designing, or rather redesigning, this powerful visage in my life. I thought for a while, imagining who I would really love for her to become.

I began with changing her attire. I gave her long, flowing white robes embroidered with flowers of every color of the rainbow. I let her hair down and softly brushed it out for her. It fell gracefully below her shoulders. I placed her outside in a beautiful garden, and as the sun shone down on her, pink cheeks appeared to replace her ashen skin. I gave her lavender oil to calm her, rose oil for love, and chocolate to give her a taste of life's sweetness. Finally, I gave her a mantra: "I forgive you, and I forgive myself." Aww . . . now, that is closer to a trusted wise woman.

There was one more piece I needed to bring into this makeover. What did her voice sound like? What could I do to replace my inner critic's strident, ever-judging voice? I thought and considered. Finally, it came to me. I would replace this Supreme Court justice with a comedian—an older, wise woman. *Who would that be?* I wondered. As I sat quietly, the voice of one person came into my mind: Joan Rivers. Perfect! Joan Rivers had a wonderful sense of humor, and always had a hilarious or at least clever comment to make about everything. Joan Rivers was my girl. I never looked back from there. My inner critic was now rebranded. I gave myself a hug and gratefully, joyfully embraced all that I was.

It took a little practice and awareness for me to implement and integrate the "being nature" of my newly minted wise woman inner critic, but I was determined to shift my internal dialogue. I held the intention to listen to this new version, and if I ever heard the voice of the old judgmental inner critic in my mind, I reminded her that she had a new role and to kindly get with the program.

Now, how can you shift your inner critic to be more like a wise, loving, maybe even humorous companion?

Here is a review of this tool for you:

- We all make mistakes. Instead of feeling bad about it, see them as avenues for further discovery.
- If you are hearing negative self-talk, decide to make a change—and make it!
- Notice how your inner critic is showing up for you.
- Rebrand your inner critic. Then consciously stick with this new, kinder voice as you integrate it into your life.
- Give yourself a hug and embrace all that you are.
- Be gentle with yourself. Please.

To be human is to "be," not to "be perfect." We may be momentarily hesitant when things don't go the way we expected or wanted. That's not really the point. The point is this: you are doing the best you can. And what are you learning in these moments of making mistakes? Your world doesn't suddenly become less meaningful at these times. The world doesn't stop spinning on its axis. You haven't broken some cardinal rule. You are not bad, wrong, or unworthy. You are *human.*

We forgive ourselves when things go differently from how we intended. It doesn't matter if it's a moment's falter or a bigger thing. We must stand for ourselves in self-love, self-worth, self-acceptance, and self-compassion, no matter what infraction we commit or think we cause. Forgiveness and self-compassion are foundational to building a sturdy, healthy, happy life with ease and joy.

We are enough. You are enough. You always were enough. Give yourself love, always.

Exercise: Ways to Release Negative Thinking Habits

How do we begin to shift from our security alarm gone awry—the voice endlessly chattering frustration, resentment, bitterness, and discomfort with ourselves—back to the healthier, more logical alarm that helps keep us safe? Here are a few tools that I have found helpful:

- *Become aware of your negative thinking patterns.* Do an assessment from a neutral place of observation. For example, *Oh, look at that. I have a pattern of thinking that things will always go wrong for me. Or, I keep hearing myself say I never finish what I start. Or, Oh, I just said, "I'll never be enough, no matter what I do."* In this step you are just becoming aware of your thinking and taking inventory of the negatives.

- *Do not complete a negative thought about yourself.* It has been an interesting and challenging practice for me to notice when I am saying something mean or harsh to myself, but it is possible to do it—that's the point. The more I catch myself with a thought that is trying to put me down, the less often such thoughts arise. Changing the thought in midstream is a way to change the brain's patterning into a healthier state.

- **Meet yourself where you are.** We are adept at ignoring, looking away, or just plain stuffing down whatever we are experiencing that does not seem or feel pleasant to us. We can easily get into the habit of looking away from ourselves when things get uncomfortable. We are so used to others criticizing our mistakes despite our best efforts, instead of being championed for our courage to try, that we get in the habit of criticizing ourselves. That criticism can quickly accelerate into self-loathing if we don't take steps to turn it around. When we face ourselves, we can step into the work of healing whatever we have been avoiding. Whatever we are experiencing in the moment and how we are processing it is information for us to use to make healthy choices about how we are going to respond.

- **Accept all of who you are.** When we accept that we have all the emotions of any human, with all their twists and turns, then we find a measure of peace. We are who we are. We are in the human experience. We are doing the best we know how. Give yourself a break and embrace all of who you are. Accept yourself and allow yourself to be you.

- **Do not judge yourself.** Move to a neutral place of being. No matter what you are up to or going through, try not to look at it through the lens of "good" or "bad," but to accept it just as "is." You know that saying "It is what it is"? It may sound trite, but when I come from a neutral, more impersonal place or perspective, I find that a far greater measure of ease and freedom shows up automatically. Dropping judgment and accepting all of who we are go hand in hand.

- **Go to the breath and keep your attention there.** Allow the body to release whatever energy you are experiencing. Breathe deeply, slowly, evenly: balance your inhale and your

THE WAY THROUGH CHRONIC PAIN

exhale. This type of conscious breathing gives the primitive part of the nervous system that is constantly monitoring for our safety the signal that we are safe.

- *Be selective in how you choose to interact in the world.* We can decide how much information we really want in our lives daily. Your choices around how much news you watch, the radio stations you listen to, what you read, the people you choose to interact with—can all affect how much negativity you experience.
- *Take responsibility: you are the decider.* When we are aware of our tendencies around negative thinking, we can choose how to act. It is our choice to continue speaking to ourselves in a degrading manner or to lovingly forgive ourselves for being the vulnerable, perfectly imperfect human that we are.

By adopting these practices, we retrain ourselves. We rewire ourselves through how we take ownership in our thinking patterns of a healthier way of living. These are simple steps, but they take practice. I practice every day and am grateful to have such a powerful way of helping myself stay on a more empowered course rather than stuck in the victim mentality of being at the mercy of negative thinking patterns.

Chapter 6

Self-Reflection Questions

Think about these questions:

- What would it be like for you to step beyond your pain for a moment and imagine your divine purpose dropping down right in front of you?
- What would it be like for you to be able to live your divine purpose every day?
- How would it feel to live full-out to your potential and

136

feel the creative fire of life inside you set on max, and on a regular basis?

- What would it be like for you to listen with your heart wide open?
- Can you allow yourself to imagine the above scenarios playing out in your life? What would it take for you to believe they are possible?

Chapter 8

Self-Reflection Questions

Eckhart Tolle talks about the pain body, where we experience past patterns of negativity, like unresolved emotions and behaviors. We all have a pain body. It is part of the human condition. It's what we do with it that determines whether we will suffer.

- Is your pain body overwhelming you?
- Are you nonreactive to your pain body?
- Can you master becoming nonreactive to your pain body?
- When you notice your pain body arising in your experience, how do you react?
- Do you feed your experience of your pain body with your reaction to it? For instance, when you feel intense sensation in your body, like a headache, do you steel yourself against it? Or do you notice it and stay as the witness to it?

Exercise: Get into the Moment

To get into the moment, pause whatever you are doing. Close your eyes if you feel safe doing so, or just look at a comfortable spot. Take three slow, even inhales and exhales. When you do this, you have entered the present moment. There is no worry here. The future is off where it lives, unwritten and unseen. The past is where it belongs, in the past.

You can also pause and sit still. Notice what you feel: sound, smell, all sensations. Just make yourself present to them. There is only here. Now. Whatever you experience is what it is. It's not good or bad. It's just what you are experiencing.

Allow yourself to rest in the present moment. When you adopt this as a practice, you will train your nervous system to sit quietly. You will break up the downward spiral of chronic pain and heal. You will more readily find peace—deep inner peace.

Through this practice of presence, you will discover one of the secrets of living a thriving life.

Exercise: Box Breathing

Box breathing is a simple focusing exercise, done in four equal parts, that retrains the nervous system to breathe properly. It helps calm the nerves and relieve the tension built up in response to stress. The result of box breathing is a sense of ease and peace in the body and quiet in the mind. When we are calm, we can more easily focus on our job or the task at hand. We make fewer mistakes. We feel more successful and therefore more fulfilled.

Also known as four-square breathing, box breathing is a simple technique that you can do any time you feel stressed. This tool is especially valuable because you can carry it with you wherever you go and use it whenever you need or want to.

This controlled, even breathing is an integral part of meditation. Box breathing can be used to help regulate the autonomic nervous system. It uses control through equal counts of four, allowing your body to become nourished by deep, even breaths. The chest and abdominal muscles also get some stimulation.

The Steps to Box Breathing
1. *Sit up straight.*
2. *Begin with a complete exhalation*, pushing in and up with your abdominal muscles to help release the last bit of used air.

3. *Inhale to a count of four.* As you begin, expand your abdomen to fill the base of your lungs, and expand your whole chest cavity as you continue to fill them. As you come into your count of four, take just a little more air in at the end, imagining you are taking it in all the way up into your collarbones.

4. *Hold the breath for a count of four.*

5. *Let the breath out to a count of four.* As you exhale, gently begin at the collarbone, deflating the chest all the way down into the abdomen, pulling in your belly at the end to push out the last of the air.

6. *Hold the breath out for a count of four.*

7. *Return to Step 1 and repeat the cycle for three to eleven minutes.*

Box Breathing Meditation

Sit comfortably and let your body feel in perfect balance. Focus your attention on your breath. Sense your breath as a quality of motion as you breathe slowly and deliberately, in and out. How does it move in different parts of your body as you breathe in a slow and steady rhythm? What is the quality of your breath as you begin this exercise? Consider that it might change as you move through this meditation.

Breathe deeply and evenly, expanding your belly as you inhale. Bring the air deep into the base of your lungs and exhale fully before your next deep and measured conscious breath. Use your abdominal muscles to help press the air out of your lungs. Do your best to keep your inhale and exhale even in duration. You are oxygenating and detoxifying your whole body in this exercise. No cell is left behind here. Repeat this slow, deep, even breathing.

As you continue to breathe, bring your attention to your heartbeat. If you cannot feel your heart pulsing throughout your body, place your finger over the pulse point on your wrist and feel it there. The heartbeat follows the breath. Continue to breathe slowly and deeply as you also notice the rhythm of your heart. Breathe. Breathe. Breathe. Now you can begin to breathe with the heartbeat. Breathe into a count of four heartbeats. Hold the breath to a count of four heartbeats. Exhale to a count of four heartbeats. Hold the breath after you exhale to a count of four heartbeats. Then inhale again to a count of four and continue breathing with the rhythm of the heart. Inhale for four, hold the breath in for four, exhale for four, hold the breath out for four, and continue.

Continue this breath meditation for three to eleven minutes. You may notice that the mind creates thoughts as you do this practice. Let the thoughts be there. Watch them if they come but do your best to not engage with them. You are not your thoughts. You are the witness of your thoughts. Let them parade in and out of your awareness. If you find that your attention wanders off with a thought that arises, just notice that you are following that thought and remember to come back to the breath and the heartbeat.

Meditation is called a practice because it is just that: practice. It doesn't matter how many times you find yourself losing focus on the breath and the heartbeat and instead follow a thought. What matters is how many times you bring your attention back to the breath and the heartbeat. That is the work and the essence of meditation. Just continue with your focus on your breath and your heartbeat the best you can. However the practice is in this moment is exactly the way it is. Be content. Breathe and feel your heartbeat.

Feel the motion and the energy of the breath. Notice how the heartbeat changes with the breath and calms as you breathe consciously. The heartbeat follows the breath. Your focus is on the breath and the beat. There is only your breath and your heart, beating to the rhythm of life itself. You are life in this moment. Breathing, beating, pulsing. Let the breath breathe you as you witness the peace in this simple moment. The breath is a wave on a great ocean of energy, and you are riding on it. Right here.

Right now. You notice a point of stillness and quietude, perhaps on the beat, or between the heartbeats, when you suspend the breath. This still point is a great listening and resting spot. We find such peace here.

You are here now in this serene moment. You did the work and brought yourself here to this place. No matter the busyness of life or how hectic things seem to get, you always have this ability to pause and breathe slowly and deeply, consciously. The character of your thoughts and emotions is reflected in the motion of your breath.

Once you learn this calm breathing pattern and practice it regularly, you will notice when the quality of your breath changes as you go through your day. It may shorten and become shallower as you rise to more urgent demands. Here, too, you can always choose to pause and adjust your breath, lengthening and deepening it to help calm you and put you in a better position to respond to what life brings you, instead of automatically reacting. The conscious breath is always ready for you as your grounding and steadying force as you experience the ebbs and flows of your day.

Please take this tool of conscious breathing with you. Put it into practice the best you can. The value of meditation is that we remain as steady as we can as we do the practice. We do our best and allow ourselves to be content with however the meditation is in that moment. We are human. This is a practice, not a perfect. As we find steadiness in the breath during our meditation practice, we can take that practice with us into real life. When we experience the ebbs and flows of our day and feel buffeted by the winds of busyness and seeming chaos out in the world, we apply our practice and find we can steady and ground ourselves. One of my favorite poems is Rudyard Kipling's "If." In it he writes, "If you can keep your head when all about you are losing theirs . . ." This meditation practice will help you "keep your head" in the unpredictable life we experience. After a while, you might find that you cannot imagine how you managed before you incorporated the tool of conscious breathing into your life.

Exercise: Left Nostril Breathing for Insomnia and Anxiety

This method of breathing helps calm the nervous system and has been found to reduce stress and anxiety in daily life. It also helps prepare the body for sleep and soothe restlessness and sleeplessness. Breathing only through the left nostril also helps curb compulsive eating habits and cravings because it activates the parasympathetic nervous system, affecting digestion, elimination, and our sleep cycles.

If your mind is racing or you just can't fall asleep, left nostril breathing is a great nonpharmaceutical remedy. I also find it helpful to sit for eleven minutes every evening just before bed and use this breathing technique to settle down at the end of the day, giving my body the signal that it's time to sleep.

Please note that in this breathing technique one inhales only through the left nostril. You can exhale out of either the left or the right side, but to get the calming benefit of this practice, you must inhale through the left side. Yoga students have reported that their sleep improved after one week of practicing this breathing technique.

The Steps to Left Nostril Breathing

Block off the right nostril with your thumb or finger and breathe in through your left nostril only. Exhale through the right nostril. Use slow, even, deep breaths in and out, fully inhaling before exhaling, and fully exhaling before inhaling again.

Repeat for three to eleven minutes.

I encourage you to incorporate this breathing technique into your daily life. Observe any changes in your general level of anxiety and in your sleeping pattern.

Exercise: Alternate Nostril Breathing to Balance the Brain and Ease Headaches

This breathing technique will calm, center, and energize you in a grounded way.

Here's the science behind alternate nostril breathing.

You may not realize the importance of your nostrils. Their power lies in the energy anatomy connected to your left and right nostril.

The left nostril is linked to the right hemisphere of the brain. Breathing through this nostril brings the abilities for calming, cooling, sensitivity, empathy, and receptivity.

The right nostril is linked to the left hemisphere of the brain. Breathing through this nostril brings warmth, alertness, higher energy, willpower, and concentration.

For example, if you find throughout the day that you are primarily using your right nostril, it may indicate that you are in a state of high alert or high stress. If you find yourself primarily a left nostril breather, there may be some signs of being overly sensitive and calm to the point of mild depression.

The key with body wellness is balance, and alternate nostril breathing helps to balance the left and right sides of our brains and bodies. Early studies show that alternate nostril breathing decreases blood pressure, increases skin conductance, and affects the heart rate.

Here are some of the benefits of alternate nostril breathing:

- Increases whole-brain fitness and function by balancing the left and right hemispheres of the brain
- Promotes a deep sense of physical, mental, and emotional well-being
- Fills the body with life-bringing oxygen and helps with detoxification
- Reduces stress and anxiety
- Brings clarity and helps focus the mind, improving concentration

The Steps to Alternate Nostril Breathing

1. Open your right hand and make a U-shape with your thumb and forefinger.
2. Block the right nostril with your thumb and inhale through your left nostril.
3. Hold the inhale briefly.
4. Block the left nostril with your forefinger and release your thumb from your right nostril.
5. Exhale through the right nostril, and as you continue to block the left nostril, inhale through the right nostril.
6. Hold the inhale briefly.
7. Block the right nostril once more and exhale through the left nostril.
8. Continue for three to five minutes.
9. Finish by inhaling deeply. Pause and hold the breath for a few seconds. Exhale and lower your hand.

Chapter 9

Exercise: Tree Meditation

Now I'm going to take you on a journey into nature and share a meditation I enjoy doing with our long-lost cousins, the trees. You might find that you are called to meditate with the waters in a stream or river, or the clouds in the sky, or the breeze: whatever calls to you from nature, you can always drop in and merge with it in a meditative state.

Please imagine that you are out in nature. This is a conscious practice for you to ground and center yourself in calmness using these five tools at the ready: the earth, the heavens, the trees, your breath, and your attention.

Sit quietly on a bench or chair or step down onto the earth itself for at least twenty minutes. Set yourself up to enter a session of being-ness. Put your attention on your sitting bones and allow your weight to rest on each of them equally. Lengthen and straighten your spine, reaching from the top of your head to the sky as you extend vertically.

Imagine that the earth is welcoming you; allow yourself to sink fully into it, no longer feeling as if you must work against the forces of gravity. You are now physically centered: your base is connected to and dropped down into the earth, and your spine is open and straight. You are a conduit between the earth and the heavens. Imagine a line going from deep in the exact center of the earth straight up to the base of your seat, up through your spine, and extending out the top of your head and into the heavens. You have attuned yourself to Great Mother Earth and Great Father Sky. So long as you open your inner ears and inner eyes, you will hear and see what they are saying to you.

The surrounding tree creatures play their role well. Standing still, going nowhere, pulsing with life, they speak a deafening silence. You gaze out to the trees in front of you with eyes somewhat out of focus. As you gaze, you are aware of your breath. The earth, tree, human, sky—we all share this air, this medium of energy. Sit quietly and breathe, in and out, slowly. You feel your attention drawn to one tree in the moment. Begin a silent communion as your eyes meet and center on the tree's presence. You are in a space of no one thought, just perception and listening intently.

The trees are experts at being exactly who and what they are. They are our teachers. They remind us that we are indeed human beings, not human doings. As you move through your day and perhaps even allow yourself to feel harried with all the doings in which we entangle ourselves, our friends the trees remind us to rest a moment and center into this place of being. There is no hastiness here, no busyness, and no sense of urgency.

So, we remember exactly who we are; we are being in this moment. The earth holds us always. Sky looks over us always. We are held between these two forces. They embrace us as we move through the Great Wheel of Life. The trees remind us to be exactly where we are and who we are, in this moment. In every moment. And as we keep our attention on being, we find that sweet spot of incomparable joy in life, sitting squarely in this present moment.

Bibliography and References

Bibliography

Introduction

Bhajan PhD, Yogi. CDs of 3 Lectures by Yogi Bhajan from *Timeless wisdom from Yogi Bhajan, PhD*. From the Yoga of awareness, from the Kundalini Yoga Lecture Series. Kundalini Research Institute. https://www.libraryofteachings.com/

McCauley, K. The neuroscience of addiction. Keynote address, From Research to Rehab: A Town Hall Meeting on Substance Use and Young People. 14 April 2016. https://www.youtube.com/watch?v=MrN58Nbl_8o

Chapter 1

Integrative Pain Center of Arizona. The long-term effects of untreated chronic pain. http://www.ipcaz.org/long-term-effects-untreated-chronic-pain/

Lee, M., Silverman, S. M., Hansen, H., Patel, V. B., & Manchikanti, L. A comprehensive review of opioid-induced hyperalgesia. *Pain Physician*. 2011 Mar–Apr;14(2):145–161. https://www.ncbi.nlm.nih.gov/pubmed/21412369/

Lenti, R. Future doctors unprepared to manage pain. *National Pain Report*. 17 October 2013. http://nationalpainreport.com/future-doctors-unprepared-manage-pain-8822008.html

McAllister, M. J. Tolerance to opioid pain medications. Institute for Chronic Pain. 10 July 2014. https://www.instituteforchronicpain.org/treating-common-pain/tolerance-to-opioid-pain-medications

Portenoy, R. K. Pain management and chemical dependency. *JAMA* 1997; 278:592–593. [PubMed]

Przekop, P. The connection between chronic pain and addiction. Recovery 2.0 Online Conference. February 2016. https://r20.com/videos/connection-chronic-pain-addiction/

Chapter 2

Przekop, P. *Conquer chronic pain: An innovative mind-body approach.* Center City, MN: Hazelden. 2015.

Chapter 3

Sullivan, M. D., Cahana, A., Derbyshire, S., & Loeser, J. D. What does it mean to call chronic pain a brain disease? *Journal of Pain.* 2013 Apr;14(4):317–322. https://www.ncbi.nlm.nih.gov/pubmed/23548483

Chapter 4

Anxiety and Depression Association of America. Facts and statistics. August 2017. https://adaa.org/about-adaa/press-room/facts-statistics

Apkarian, A. V. The brain in chronic pain: Clinical implications. *Pain Management* 2011 Nov 1;1(6):577–586. https://www.ncbi.nlm.nih.gov/pmc/articles/PMC3226814/

Canadian Agency for Drugs and Technologies in Health. Short- and long-term use of benzodiazepines in patients with generalized anxiety disorders: A review of guidelines. *Rapid Response Report: Summary with Critical Appraisal.* 28 July 2014. https://www.ncbi.nlm.nih.gov/pubmedhealth/PMH0070441/

Gladding, R. This is your brain on meditation. *Psychology Today.* 22 May 2013. https://www.psychologytoday.com/blog/use-your-mind-change-your-brain/201305/is-your-brain-meditation

Kipp, E. I searched for a cure for chronic pain and found the pushers from hell instead. 11 July 2016. https://elizabeth-kipp.com/i-searched-for-a-cure-for-chronic-pain-found-the-pushers-from-hell-instead/

———. *Calm anxiety and panic with box breathing.* 2017. https://vimeo.com/232151897

Mayo Clinic Staff. Anxiety: Symptoms and causes. August 2017. https://www.mayoclinic.org/diseases-conditions/anxiety/symptoms-causes/syc-20350961

———. Diseases and conditions: Phantom pain. 3 December 2014. https://www.mayoclinic.org/diseases-conditions/phantom-pain/basics/definition/CON-20023268

National Institute of Mental Health. Despite risks, benzodiazepine use highest in older people: National Institutes of Health–supported study examines prescribing patterns. Press release. 17 December 2014. https://www.nimh.nih.gov/news/science-news/2014/despite-risks-benzodiazepine-use-highest-in-older-people.shtml

Newton, J. Health Beyond Belief. http://healthbeyondbelief.com/

Northwestern University. Why chronic pain is all in your head: Early brain changes predict which patients develop chronic pain. *ScienceDaily.* 1 July 2012. https://www.sciencedaily.com/releases/2012/07/120701191611.htm

Przekop, P. *Conquer chronic pain: An innovative mind-body approach.* Center City, MN: Hazelden. 2015.

PubMed Health. Irritable bowel syndrome (IBS). NIH—National Cancer Institute. https://www.ncbi.nlm.nih.gov/pubmedhealth/PMHT0024780/

Chapter 5

Ahmed, A. K. Brain activity shifts as pain becomes chronic. *Pain Research Forum.* 8 October 2013. http://www.painresearchforum.org/news/32409-brain-activity-shifts-pain-becomes-chronic

Dispenza, Joe. *Breaking the habit of being yourself: How to lose your mind and create a new one.* Carlsbad, CA: Hay House. 2012.

———. *Evolve your brain.* Deerfield Beach, FL: Health Communication. 2007.

Gebhart, G. F. *Scientific issues of pain and distress. Definition of pain and distress and reporting requirements for laboratory animals: Proceedings of the workshop held June 22, 2000.* Washington, DC: National Academies Press. https://www.ncbi.nlm.nih.gov/books/NBK99533/

Graybiel, A. M., Barnes, T. D., Kubota, Y., Hu, D., & Jin, D. Z. Activity of striatal neurons reflects dynamic encoding and recoding of procedural memories. *Nature.* 2005 Oct 20;437(7062):1158–1161. https://www.ncbi.nlm.nih.gov/pubmed/16237445

Integrative Pain Center of Arizona. The long-term effects of untreated chronic pain. http://www.ipcaz.org/long-term-effects-untreated-chronic-pain/

Lieberman, M. D. *Social: Why our brains are wired to connect.* New York, NY: Crown, 2013.

National Center for Biotechnology Information. Hypervigilance. Mental or behavioral dysfunction. https://www.ncbi.nlm.nih.gov/medgen/452297

Porges, S. W. *The polyvagal theory: Neurophysiological foundations of emotions, attachment, communication, and self-regulation* (Norton Series on Interpersonal Neurobiology). New York, NY: W. W. Norton. 2011.

Przekop, P. *Conquer chronic pain: An innovative mind-body approach.* Center City, MN: Hazelden. 2015.

Rosen, T. Overcoming the four aggravations. *The Daily Love.* 19 June 2011. http://thedailylove.com/the-four-aggravations/

Chapter 6

Flockhart, D. T. T., Wassenaar, L. I., et al. Tracking multi-generational colonization of the breeding grounds by monarch butterflies in eastern North America. Proceedings of the Royal Society B. 7 August 2013. http://rspb.royalsocietypublishing.org/content/280/1768/20131087

Livingston, S. Does a tiny sea creature hold the key to heart regeneration? *University of Florida News.* 26 June 2017. http://news.ufl.edu/articles/2017/06/does-a-tiny-sea-creature-hold-the-key-to-heart-regeneration.php

Lumley, M. A., Cohen, J. L., Borszcz, G. S., et al. Pain and emotion: A biopsychosocial review of recent research *Journal of Clinical Psychology.* 2011 Sept;67(9):942–968. https://www.ncbi.nlm.nih.gov/pmc/articles/PMC3152687/

McEwen, B. S. Stressed or stressed out: What's the difference? *Journal of Psychiatry and Neuroscience.* 2005 Sep;30(5): 315–318. https://www.ncbi.nlm.nih.gov/pmc/articles/PMC1197275/

Newton, J. Health Beyond Belief. http://healthbeyondbelief.com/

NIH. *Genetic information and the workplace report.* National Institutes of Health (NIH): ELSI Program Report. National Human Genome Research Institute. 20 January 1998. https://www.genome.gov/10001732/

USDA Forest Service. Migration and overwintering. https://www.fs.fed.us/wildflowers/pollinators/Monarch_Butterfly/migration/

Wills, H. The art of well-being and higher consciousness. http://www.howardwills.com/

Chapter 7

Alcoholics Anonymous. *Twelve steps and twelve traditions.* New York, NY: AA World Services. 2013.

Chronic Pain Anonymous. *Recipe for recovery: A guide to the twelve steps of Chronic Pain Anonymous.* Scottsdale, AZ: Chronic Pain Anonymous Service Board. 2015. http://chronicpainanonymous.org

Narcotics Anonymous. *Basic text: Narcotics anonymous.* Van Nuys, CA: NAWS. 2009. https://www.na.org/

Chapter 8

Aravind Kumar, R., Ramaprabha, P., & Bhuvaneswari, T. Effect of Nadi Shodhana Paranayma on cardiovascular parameters among first year MBBS students. *International Research Journal of Pharmaceutical and Applied Sciences.* 2013;3(4):103–106. http://www.irjpas.com/File_Folder/IRJPAS%203(4)103-106.pdf

Divine, M. The big four of mental toughness, part 2. SEALFIT. 19 April 2012. https://sealfit.com/the-big-4-of-mental-toughness-part-2/

Hawkins, D. R. *Recovery and healing.* Sedona, AZ: Veritas. 2009.

Holcombe, K. Breathe easy: Relax with Pranayama. *Yoga Journal.* 15 June 2012. https://www.yogajournal.com/practice/healing-breath

Kabat-Zinn, J., Lipworth, L., & Burney, R. The clinical use of mindfulness meditation for the self-regulation of chronic pain. *Journal of Behavioral Medicine.* 1985 Jun;8(2):163–90. https://www.ncbi.nlm.nih.gov/pubmed/3897551

Raghuraj, P., & Telles, S. Immediate effect of specific nostril manipulating yoga breathing practices on autonomic and respiratory variables. *Applied Psychophysiology Biofeedback.* 2008 Jun;33(2):65–75. https://www.ncbi.nlm.nih.gov/pubmed/18347974

Riordan, A. Yoga tips for insomnia. Purusha Healing Yoga. 13 September 2012. http://purushahealingyoga.com/kundalini-yoga-tips-for-insomnia.html

Saraswati, Swami S. *Asana Pranayama Mudra Bandha.* 2nd ed. Bihar, India: Bihar Yoga Bharati. 1996. pp. 379–385.

Sullivan, M. D., Cahana, A., Derbyshire, S., & Loeser, J. D. What does it mean to call pain a brain disease? *Journal of Pain.* 2013 Apr:14(40:317–22. https://www.ncbi.nlm.nih.gov/pubmed/23548483

Swami, J. Traditional yoga and meditation of the Himalayan masters. http://www.swamij.com/yoga-sutras-30103.htm

Taylor, T. Lungs. InnerBody.com. http://www.innerbody.com/anatomy/respiratory/lungs#full-description

3HO. Pranayam techniques: Left and right nostril breathing. 3HO.org https://www.3ho.org/kundalini-yoga/pranayam/pranayam-techniques/left-and-right-nostril-breathing

Chapter 9

AASM. Health sleep habits. *Sleep Education.* AASM. 9 February 2017. http://www.sleepeducation.org/essentials-in-sleep/healthy-sleep-habits

Goglia, P. L. *Turn up the heat: Unlock the fat-burning power of your metabolism.* North Charleston, SC: BookSurge. 2009.

Hartranft, C. *The yoga-sutra of Patanjali: A new translation with commentary.* Shambhala Classics. Boulder, CO: Shambhala. 2003.

Yogananda, P. *The autobiography of a yogi.* Self-Realization Fellowship. Los Angeles, CA. 1994.

Chapter 10

Alvarez, G. G., & Ayas, N. T. The impact of daily sleep duration on health: A review of the literature. *Progress in Cardiovascular Nursing,* 9(2). Spring 2004. pp. 56–59. http://onlinelibrary.wiley.com/wol1/doi/10.1111/j.0889-7204.2004.02422.x/full

Bratman, G. N., Hamilton, J. P., Hahn, K. S., Daily, G. C., & Gross, J. J. Nature experience reduces rumination and subgenual prefrontal cortex activation. Proceedings of the National Academies of Sciences. July 2015. 112 (28) 8567–8572. https://doi.org/10.1073/pnas.1510459112

Chronic Pain Anonymous. https://chronicpainanonymous.org/

Emmons, R. A., & McCullough, M. E. Counting blessings versus burdens: An experimental investigation of gratitude and subjective well-being in daily life. *Journal of Personality and Social Psychology, 84(2)*. 2003. pp. 377–389. https://greatergood.berkeley.edu/images/application_uploads/Emmons-CountingBlessings.pdf

Fox, G. R., Kaplan, J., Damasio, H., & Damasio, A. Neural correlates of gratitude. *Frontiers in Psychology*. Sept 2015; (6) 1491. https://www.ncbi.nlm.nih.gov/pmc/articles/PMC4588123/

Narcotics Anonymous. https://www.na.org/

Lutz, A., Brefczynski-Lewis, J., Johnstone, T., & Davidson, R. J. Regulation of the neural circuitry of emotion by compassion meditation: Effects of meditative expertise. *PLoS One*. 2008;3(3) doi: 10.1371/journal.pone.0001897. https://www.ncbi.nlm.nih.gov/pmc/articles/PMC2267490/

Rakic, P. Neurogenesis in adult primate neocortex: An evaluation of the evidence. *Nature Reviews Neuroscience, 3*(1);65–71. January 2002. https://www.ncbi.nlm.nih.gov/pubmed/11823806

Recovery 2.0. https://r20.com/

Refuge Recovery. https://www.refugerecovery.org/

Satchidananada, Sri Swami. *The yoga sutras of Patanjali.* Reprint ed. Buckingham, VA: Integral Yoga Publications. 14 September 2012. https://www.amazon.com/Yoga-Sutras-Patanjali-Swami-Satchidananda/dp/1938477073

SMART Recovery. https://www.smartrecovery.org/

3HO. The 5 sutras of the Aquarian age. 3HO. https://www.3ho.org/3ho-lifestyle/5-sutras-aquarian-age

Yoga 12-Step Recovery (Y12SR). http://y12sr.com/

Chapter 11

Przekop, P. Personal communication. May 2017.

References

Chronic Pain Anonymous. https://chronicpainanonymous.org/

Chopra, D. *The return of Merlin*. New York, NY: Ballantine Books. 1996.

Hazelden Betty Ford Foundation. The Betty Ford Center, Rancho Mirage, CA 92270. http://www.hazeldenbettyford.org/locations/betty-ford-center-rancho-mirage

Kundalini Research Institute. http://kundaliniresearchinstitute.org/

McCauley, K. *Addiction: New understanding, fresh hope, real healing*. Salt Lake City, UT: Institute for Addiction Study. 2007.

Newton, J. Health Beyond Belief. http://healthbeyondbelief.com/

Porges, S. W. *The polyvagal theory: Neurophysiological foundations of emotions, attachment, communication, and self-regulation* (Norton Series on Interpersonal Neurobiology). New York, NY: W. W. Norton. 2011.

Przekop, P. *Conquer chronic pain: An innovative mind-body approach*. Center City, MN: Hazelden. 2015.

Singer, M. *The untethered soul: The journey beyond yourself*. Oakland, CA: New Harbinger Publications/Noetic Books. 2007.

Tolle, E. *The power of now*. Novato, CA: New World Library. 2010.

Yogananda, P. *The autobiography of a yogi*. Self-Realization Fellowship. Los Angeles, CA. 1994.

Acknowledgments

This book would not have been possible without the guidance and encouragement of Peter Przekop, John Newton, Tommy Rosen, Larry Kipp, Mastin Kipp, Tim Lawrence, Jay Remer, Sandy Bassett, Guru Prem Singh Khalsa, Mary Sankus, Dan Schamle, Tim Shirley, Cheryl Larson, Tiffany Walter, Allison Zschiesche, Etti Palitz, Robert Anderson, Debbie Perret, Robyn M Fritz, Laurel Robinson, Robert Lanphear, Greg Cohane, and countless others who helped me find my way through to crack the code to chronic pain and discover a thriving life.

About the Author

Elizabeth R. Kipp, BS, RYT/IKYTA, is a best-selling author, Certified Recovery Coach (Recovery 2.0), Ancestral Clearing Practitioner, Bilateral EFT/Tapping Practitioner, and certified Kundalini Yoga Teacher (RYT/IKYTA/Yoga Alliance). She specializes in stress and chronic pain management. Elizabeth has a diverse background in plant science, agriculture, ecology, environmental studies, and remote sensing. She holds a Bachelor of Science degree in plant science from the University of Delaware with an emphasis on soil science and plant ecology, and pursued a master of science degree in environmental studies at the University of Kansas with an emphasis on remote sensing, ecology, and environmental resource analysis. She has done basic and applied research and has authored and co-authored a number of peer-reviewed research papers.

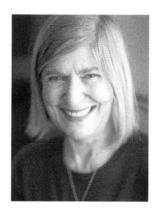

Elizabeth Kipp is a longtime seeker of truths with a foot in both the spiritual and scientific worlds. Her life experiences and training enable her to bridge the gap between these two worlds.

In the months after the birth of her son in 1982, Elizabeth's burgeoning professional career was cut short by the emergence of a structural weakness in her low spine. She spent the next thirty-one years in and out of hospitals in pursuit of a way to stabilize her spine and find freedom from the persistent pain from an old injury.

Her deep connection to the spiritual world supported her through multiple surgeries, decades of prescribed medications, and a long, persistent search for modalities that would help her heal. In 2015 Elizabeth entered a pain management program where she was able to free herself of the chronic pain cycle and find a way to live a life free of suffering.

Now in recovery, Elizabeth helps people step into the power of their own healing. She has turned her attention as a patient advocate in service to the alarmingly high number of people who suffer from or are in recovery from chronic pain.

Printed in Great Britain
by Amazon